Outis:
A Nursing Elegy

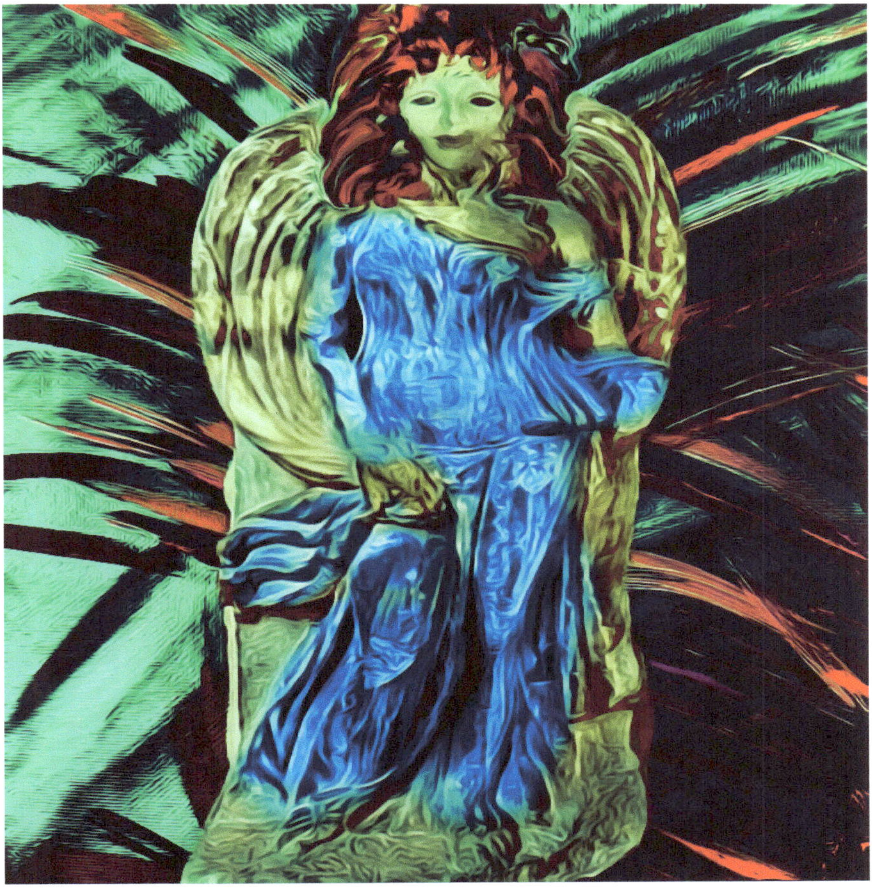

Kit Ludlow

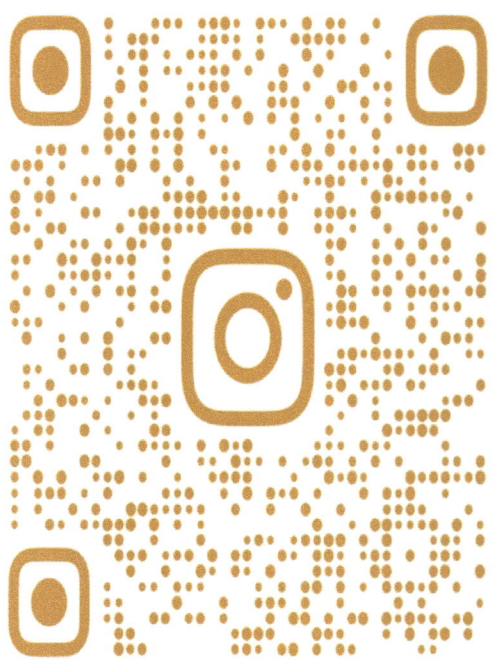

@KITLUDLOW

Copyright © Dec 2021 Kit Ludlow

All rights reserved.

ISBN: 9798786654791

FOR PERSEPHONE

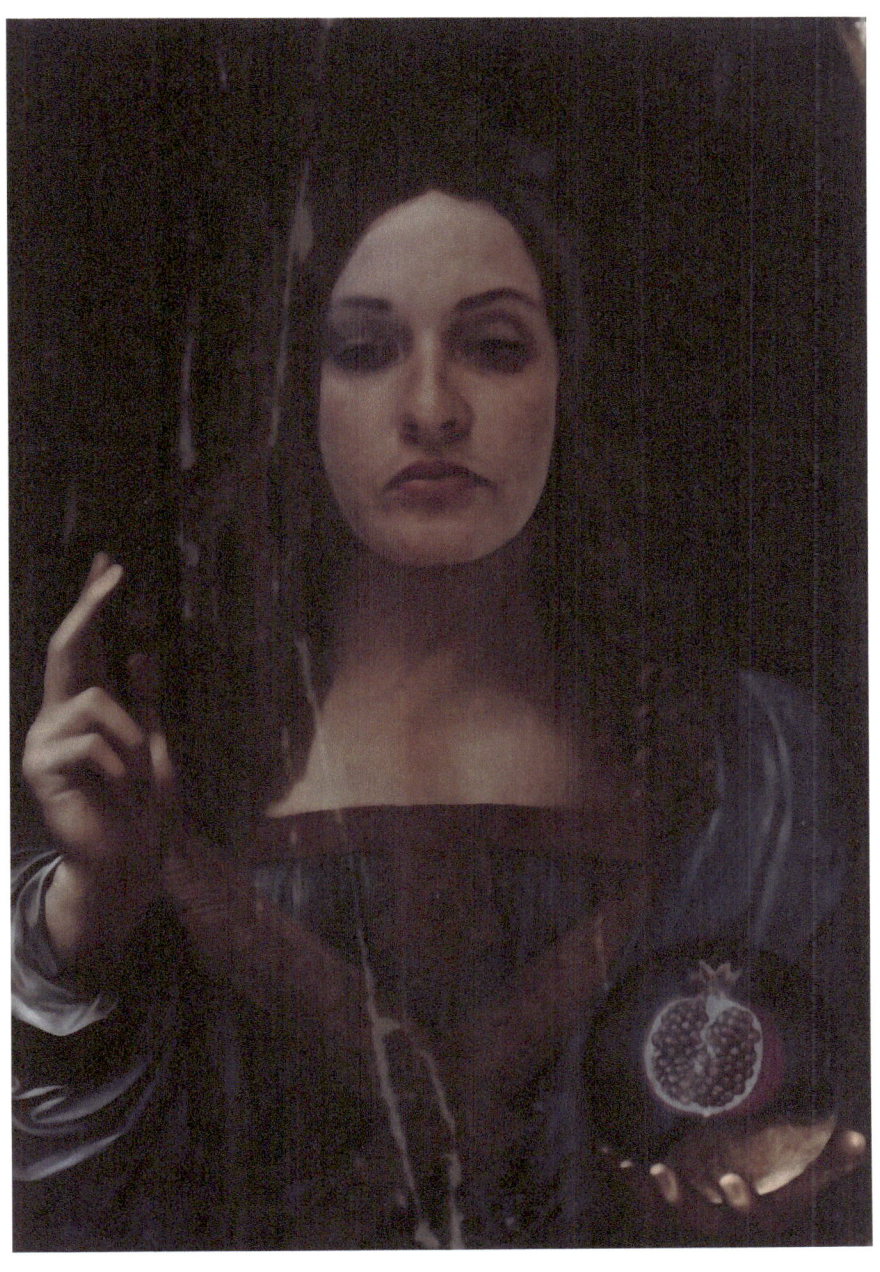

Outis: A Nursing Elegy

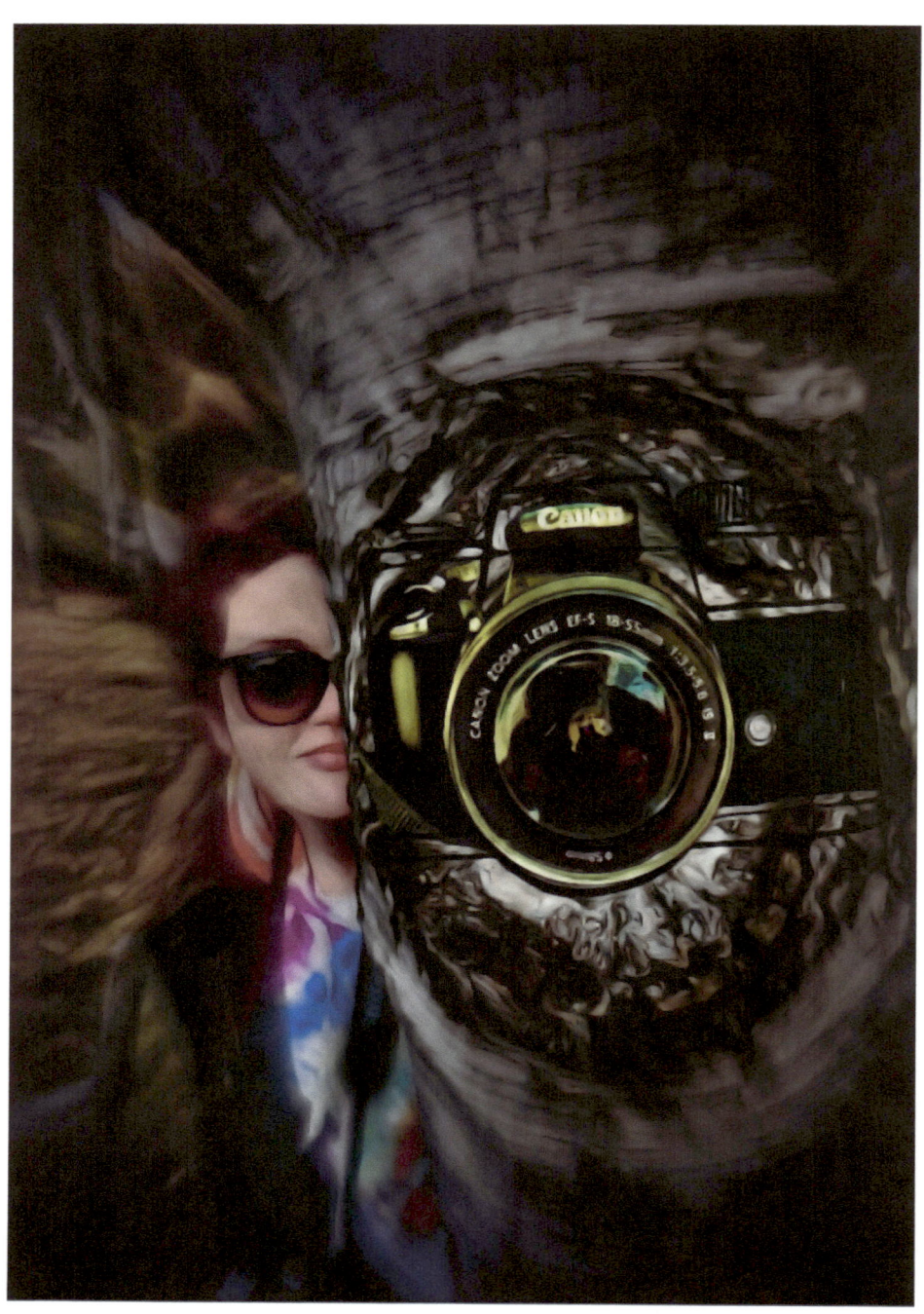

MERRY CHRISTMAS

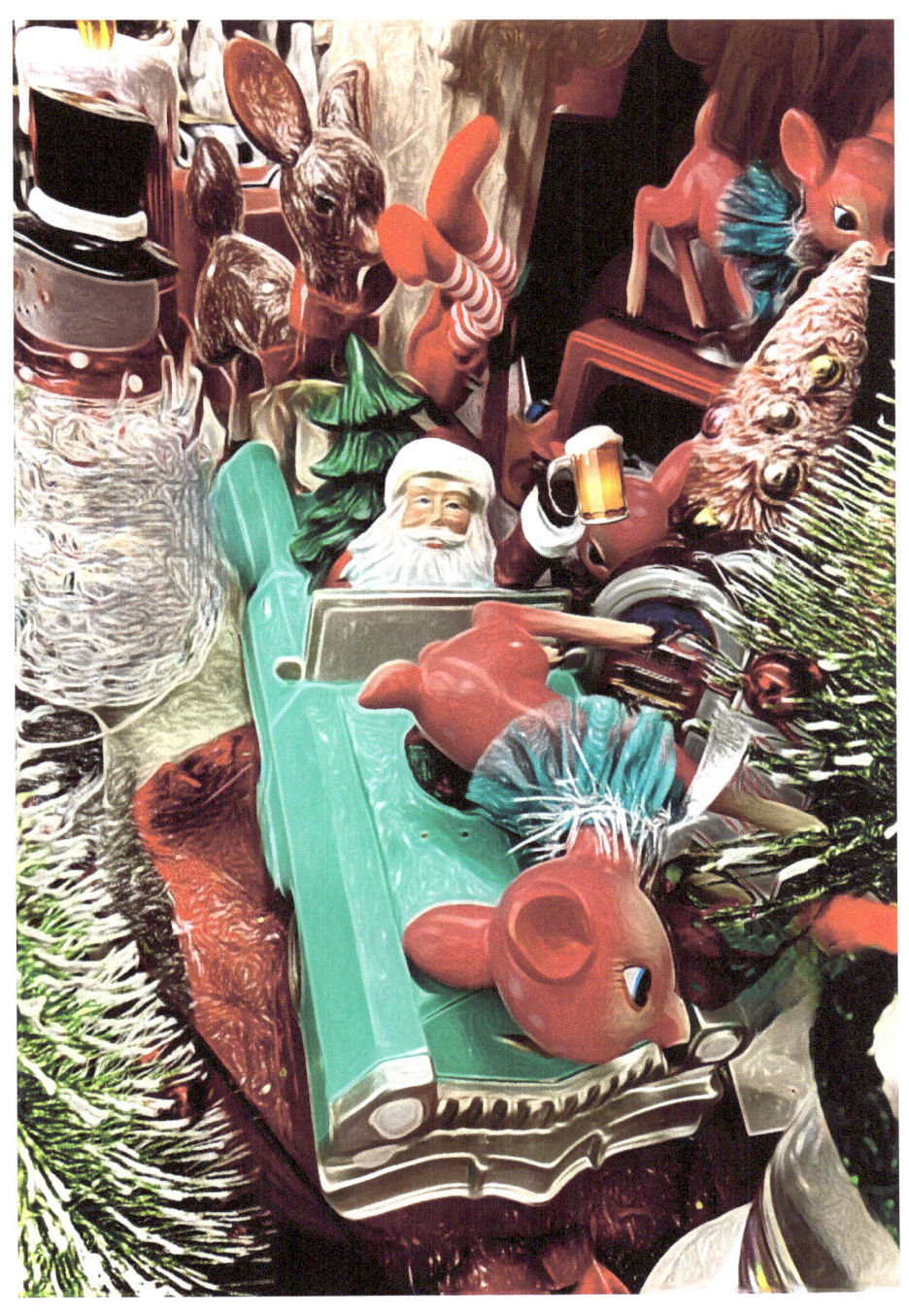

PROLOGUE

Books, the museum.
                Galleries, my mind.
The art echoes thoughts.
                Emotion fuels life,
And how I feel all-
                The flutter of wings-
The chaos of wind-
                Green shifts to scarlet,
Then a yellowed fall-
                The cold in my bones-
The dwindling lights-
                The twilight carving-
The hauntings of death. . .
                Real or imagined?
I have measured souls
                By the weights of breaths.
They weigh
        heavier
            than
                21 grams.
I've Inhaled last gasps,
                Felt a final pulse,
Charted it all down
                For grant and study.
The grotesque **shadows**
                Wherever I go.
That's why I'm Hades,
                Death is Persephone,
And all else are shades in the underworld. . .

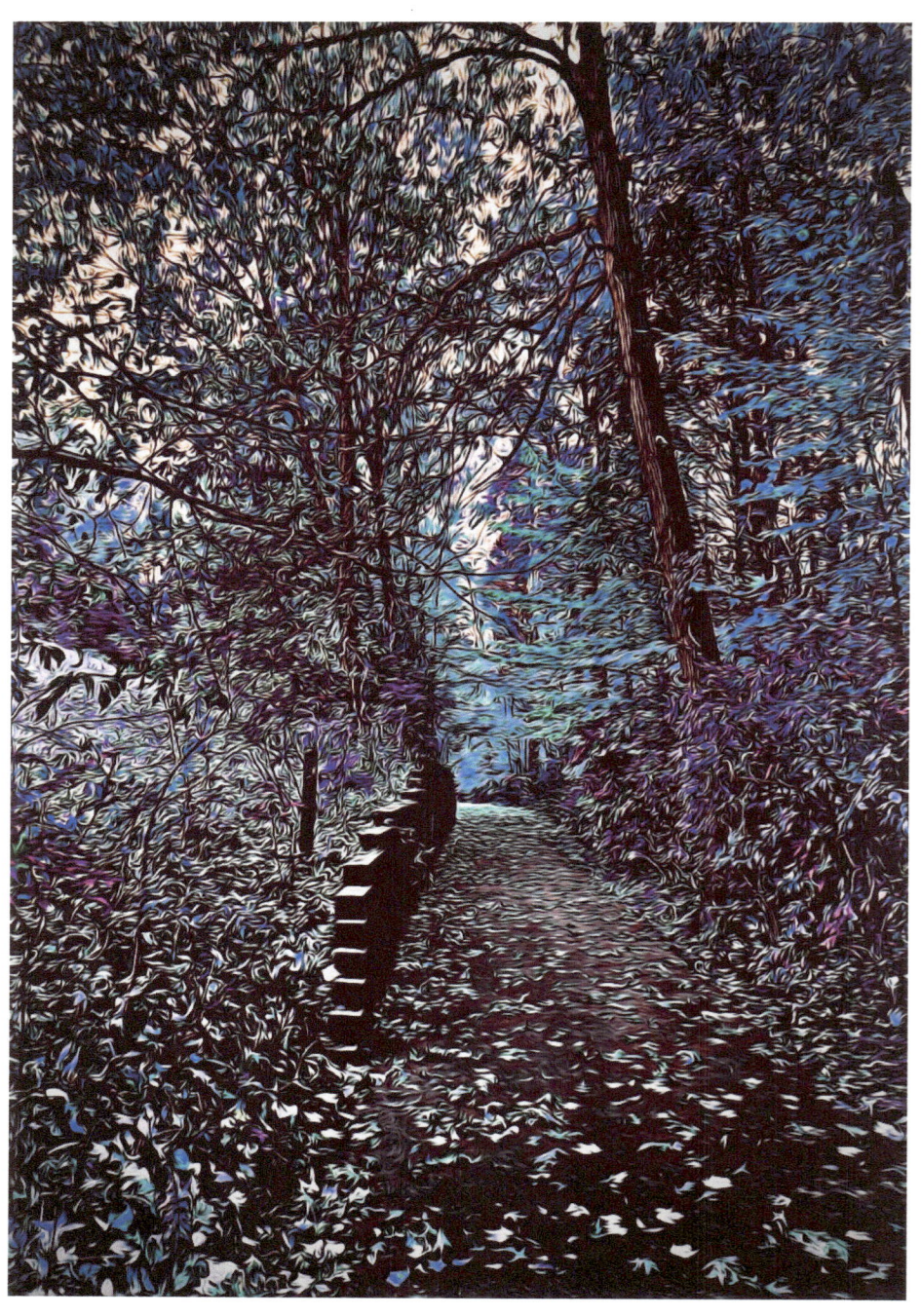

The autumn rain dripping from the shedding boughs

Outis: A Nursing Elegy

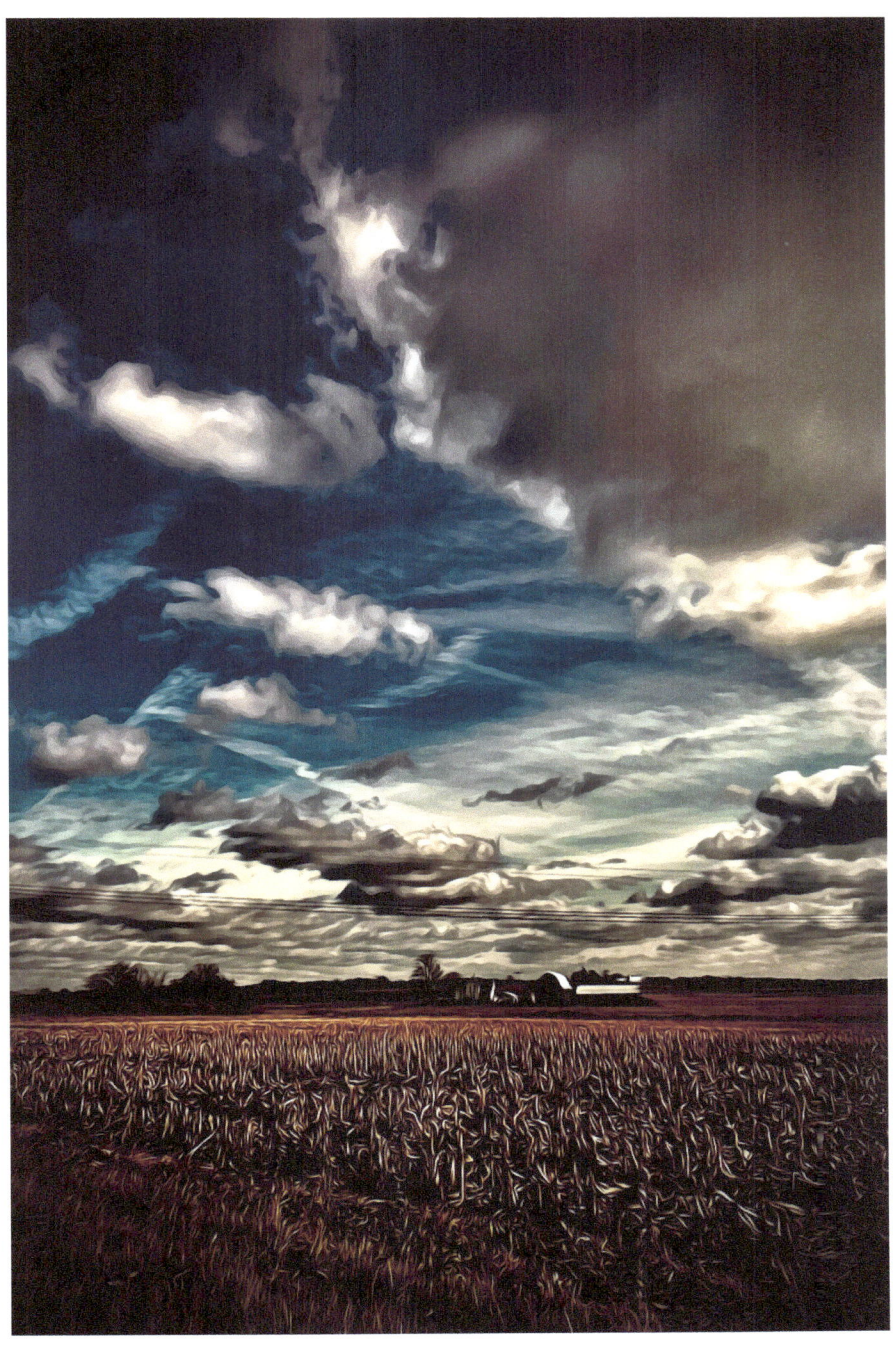

Waving to and fro from winds whirling up a cold-

Outis: A Nursing Elegy

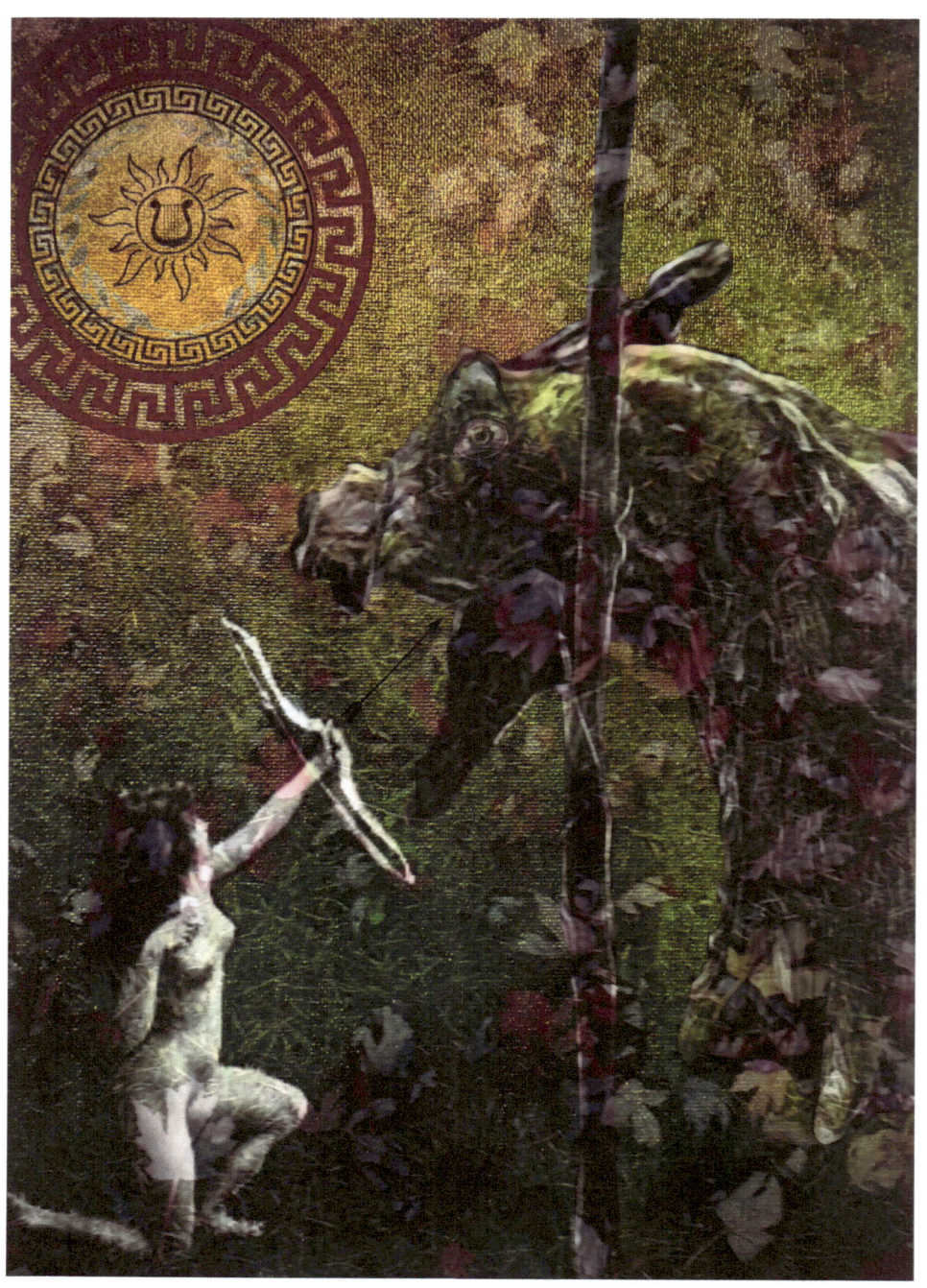

A haiku to decipher nature's fickle vows.

Outis: A Nursing Elegy

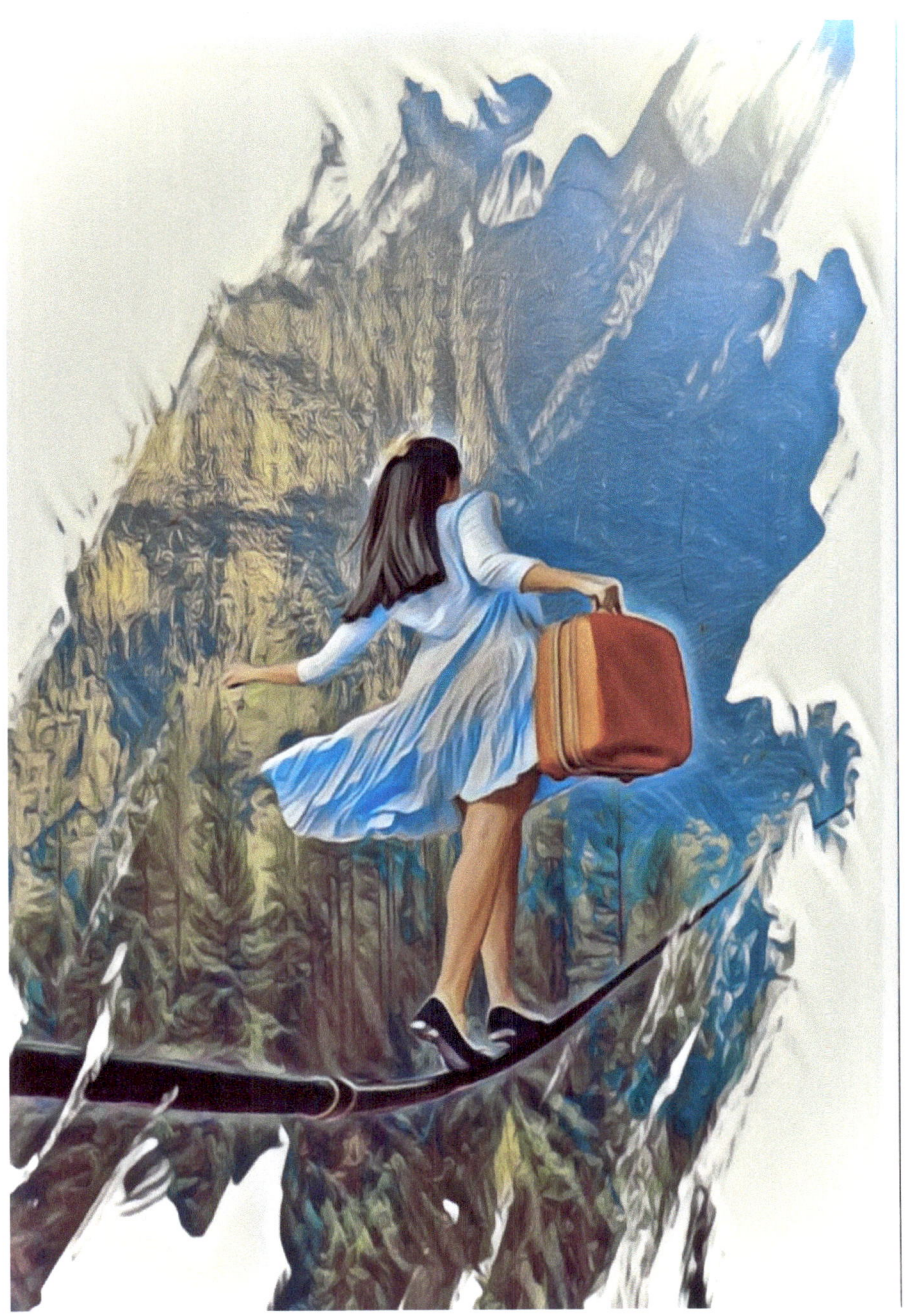

Home-lost travelers tread through the trials of trails.

Outis: A Nursing Elegy

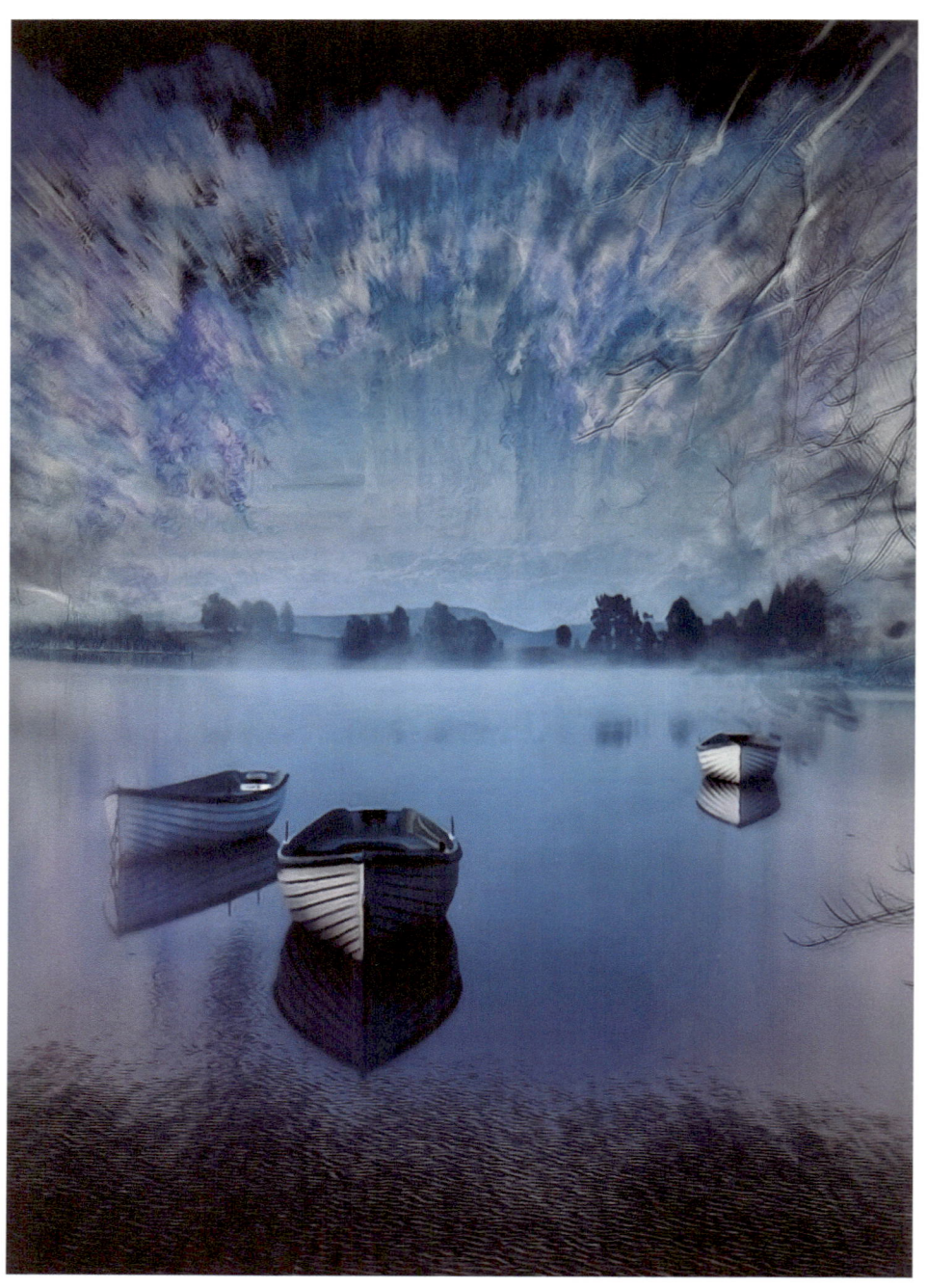

Tales tallied to tell to those that never patrolled

Outis: A Nursing Elegy

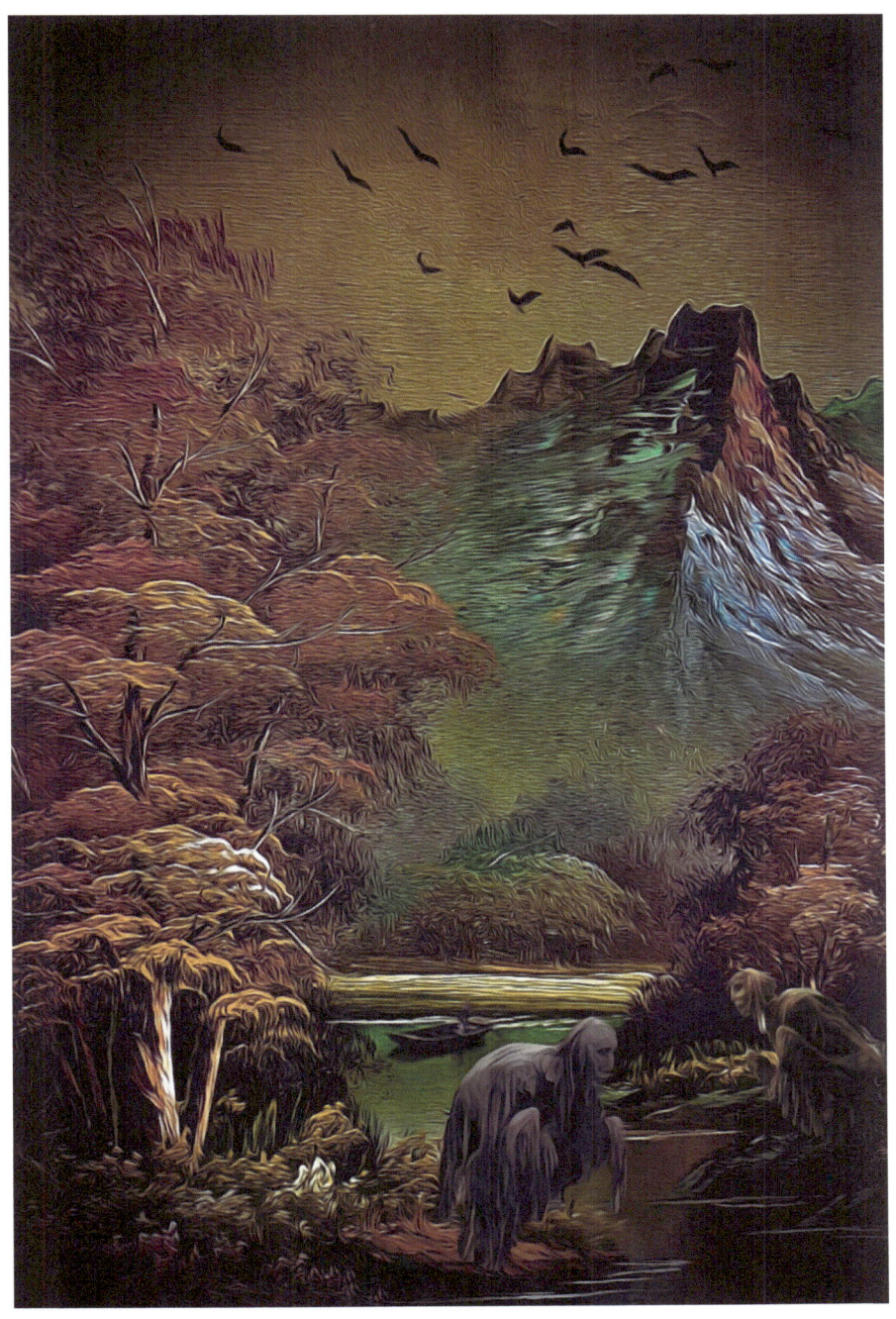

Like a ship with no sails among the gush of gales.

Outis: A Nursing Elegy

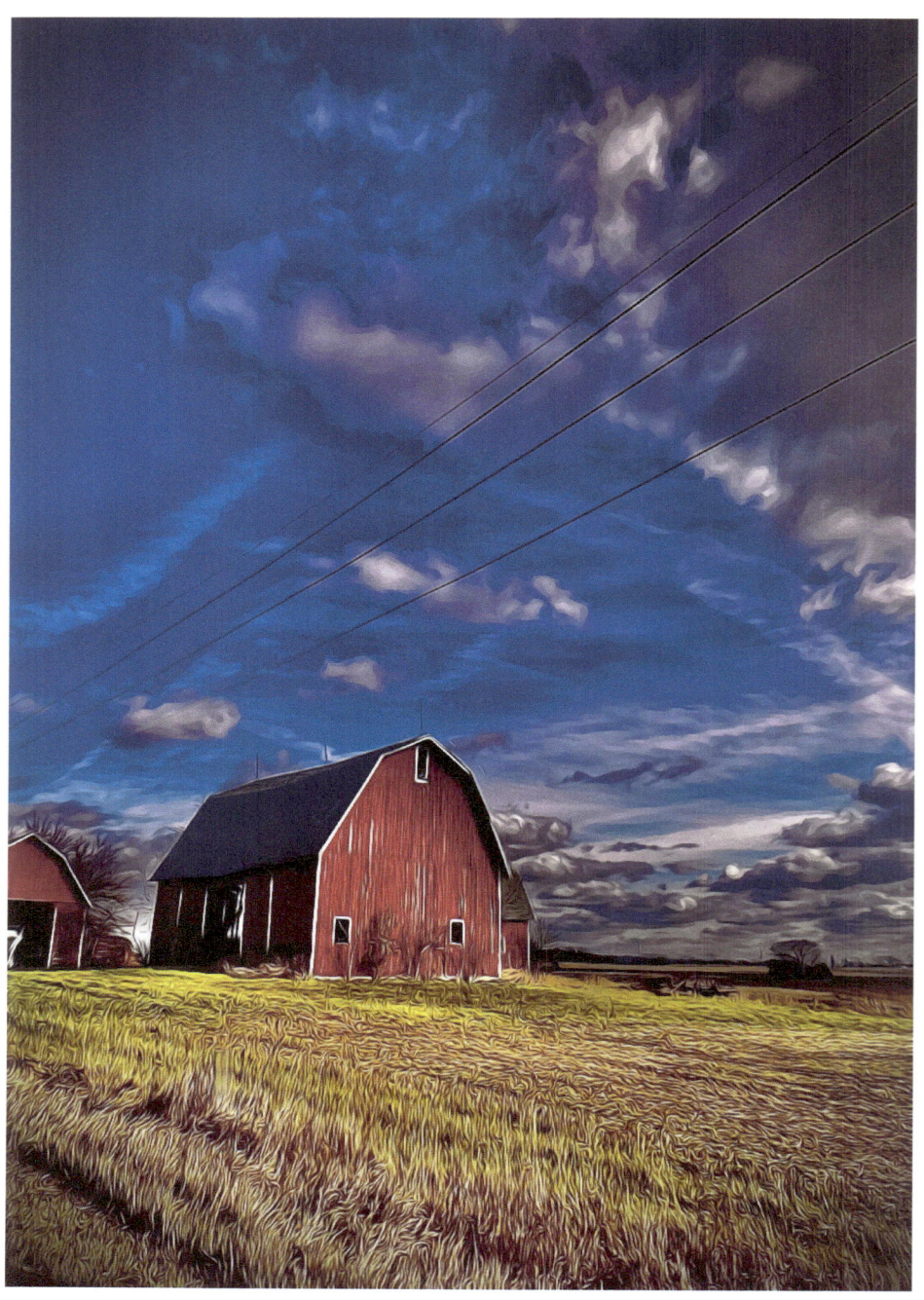

Winding breezes winnow through the harvest of grain. . .

Outis: A Nursing Elegy

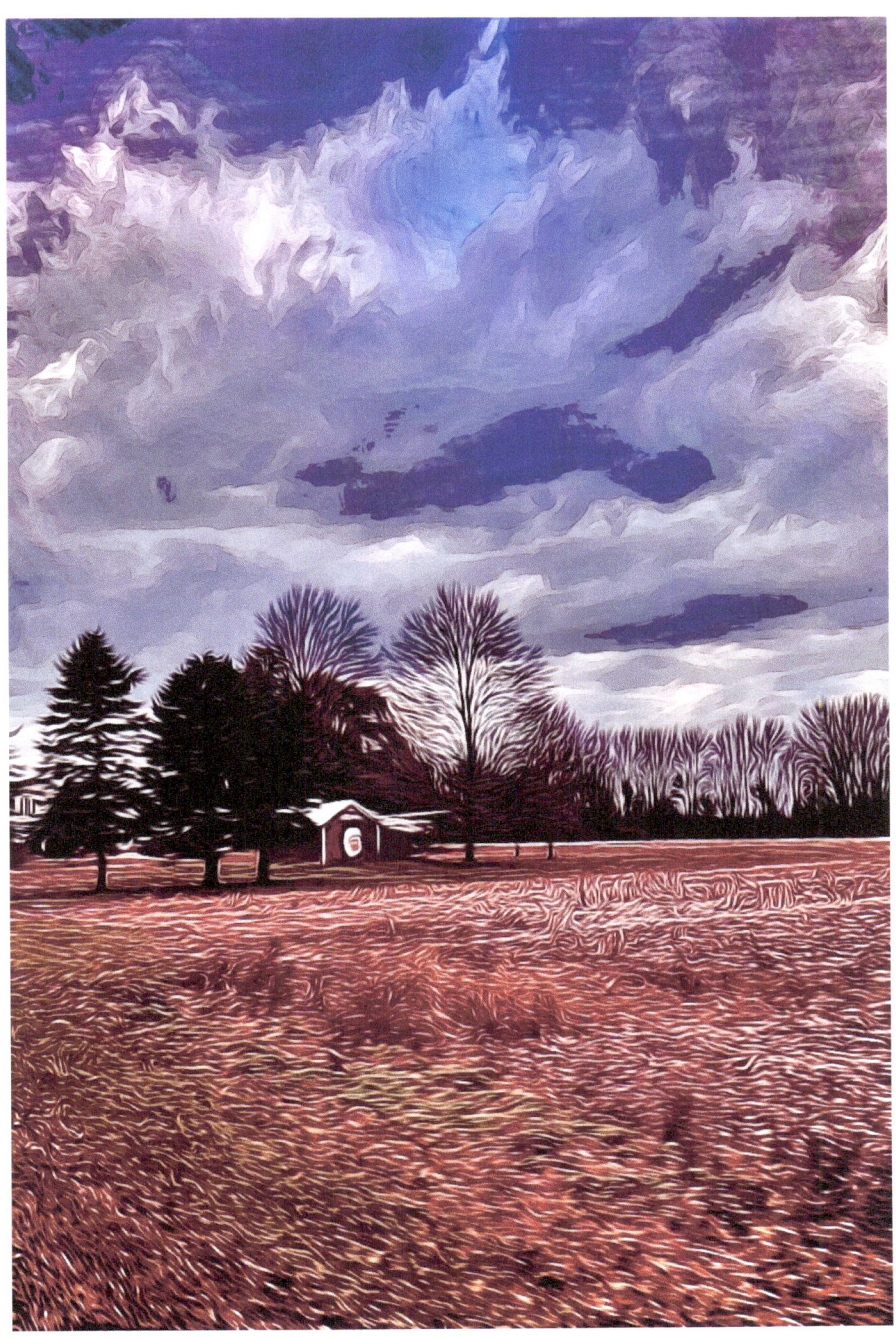

Haystacks dance upon stubble-fields with hedge witches.

Outis: A Nursing Elegy

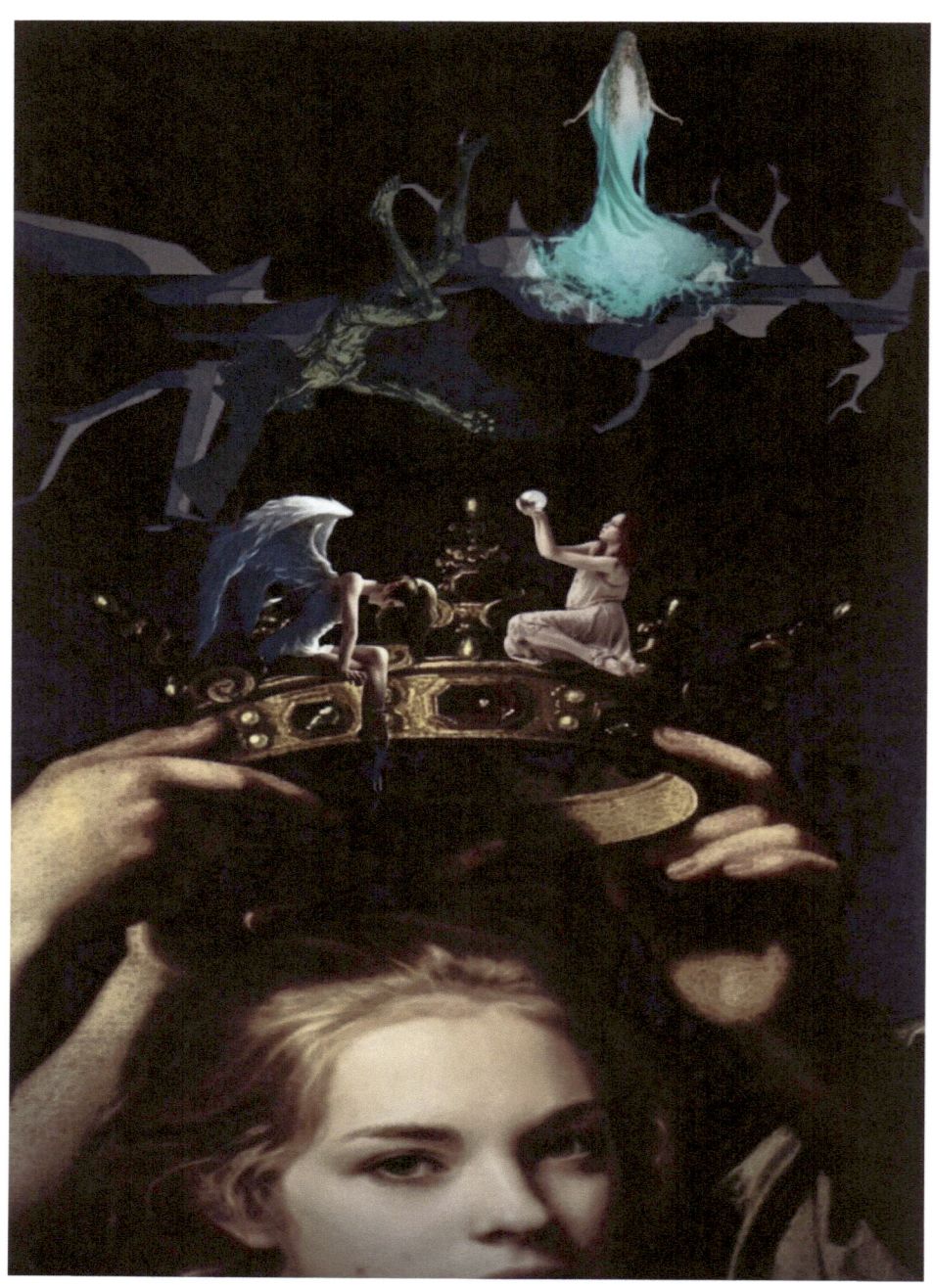

Breaths conspire, exhale the sacred name to a pain,

Outis: A Nursing Elegy

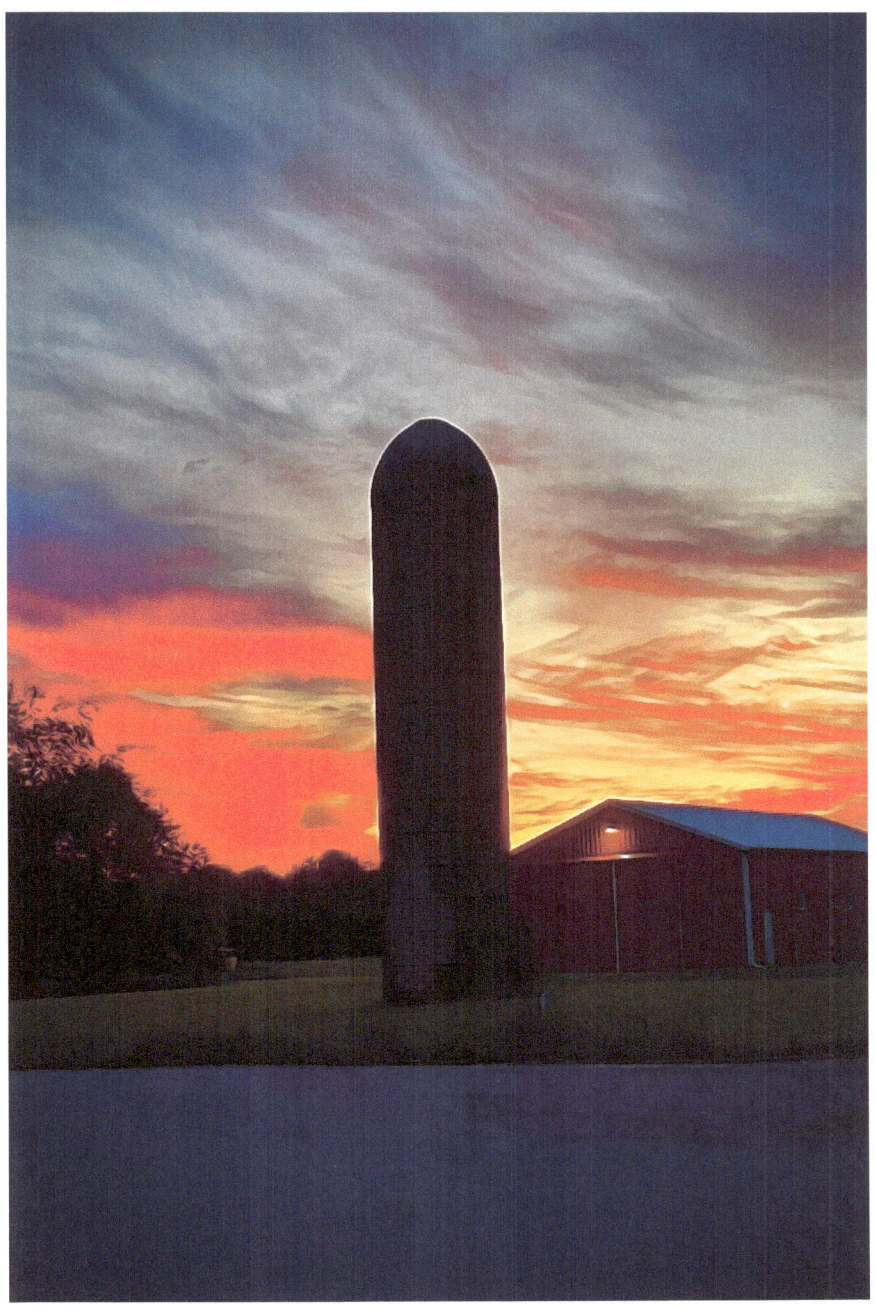

The ache of change. . .

Outis: A Nursing Elegy

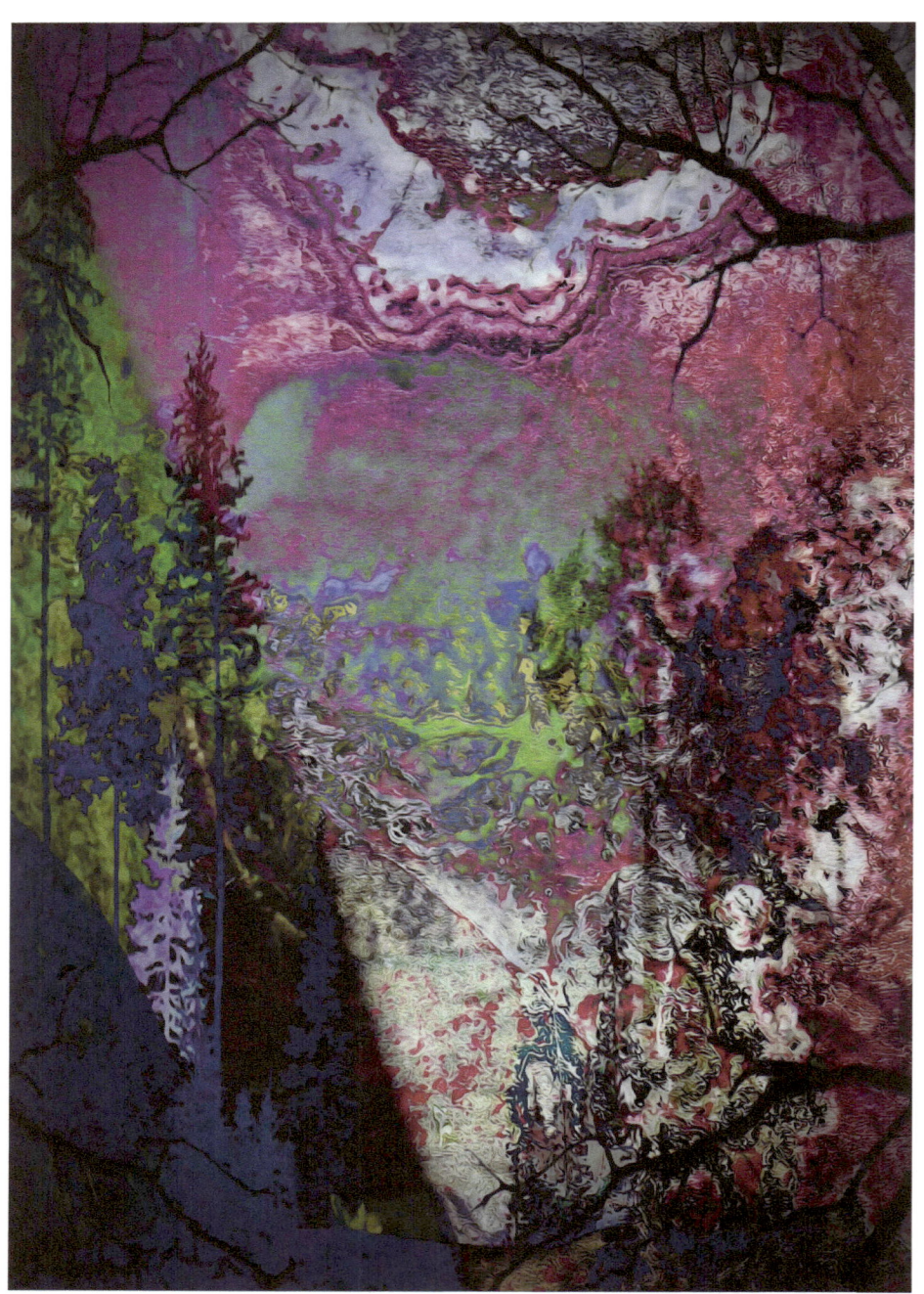

Spring promises broken by truth. . .

Outis: A Nursing Elegy

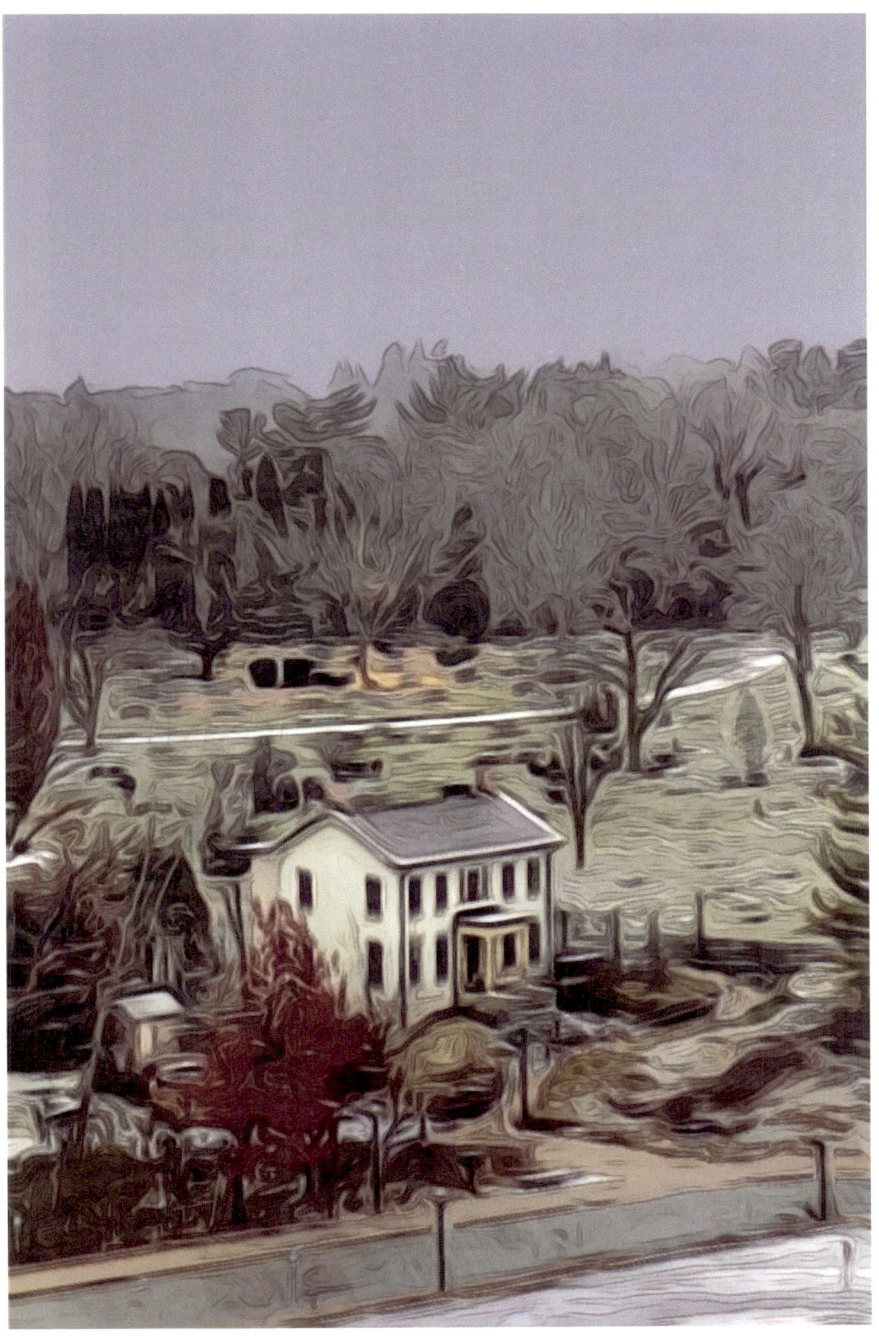

All doesn't bloom for beauty or live out its riches.

Outis: A Nursing Elegy

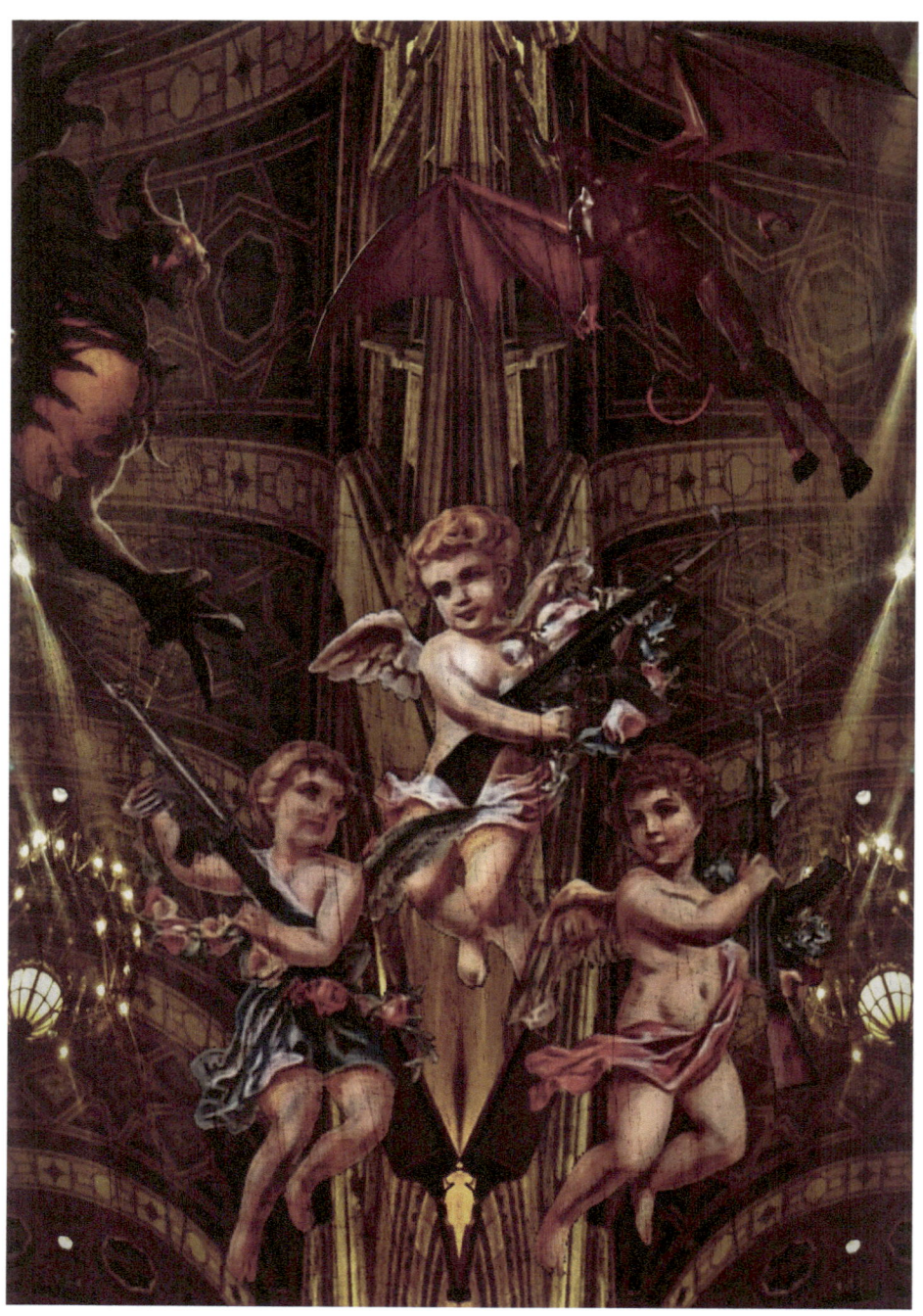

The sickness of youth can fester from well-dug roots

Outis: A Nursing Elegy

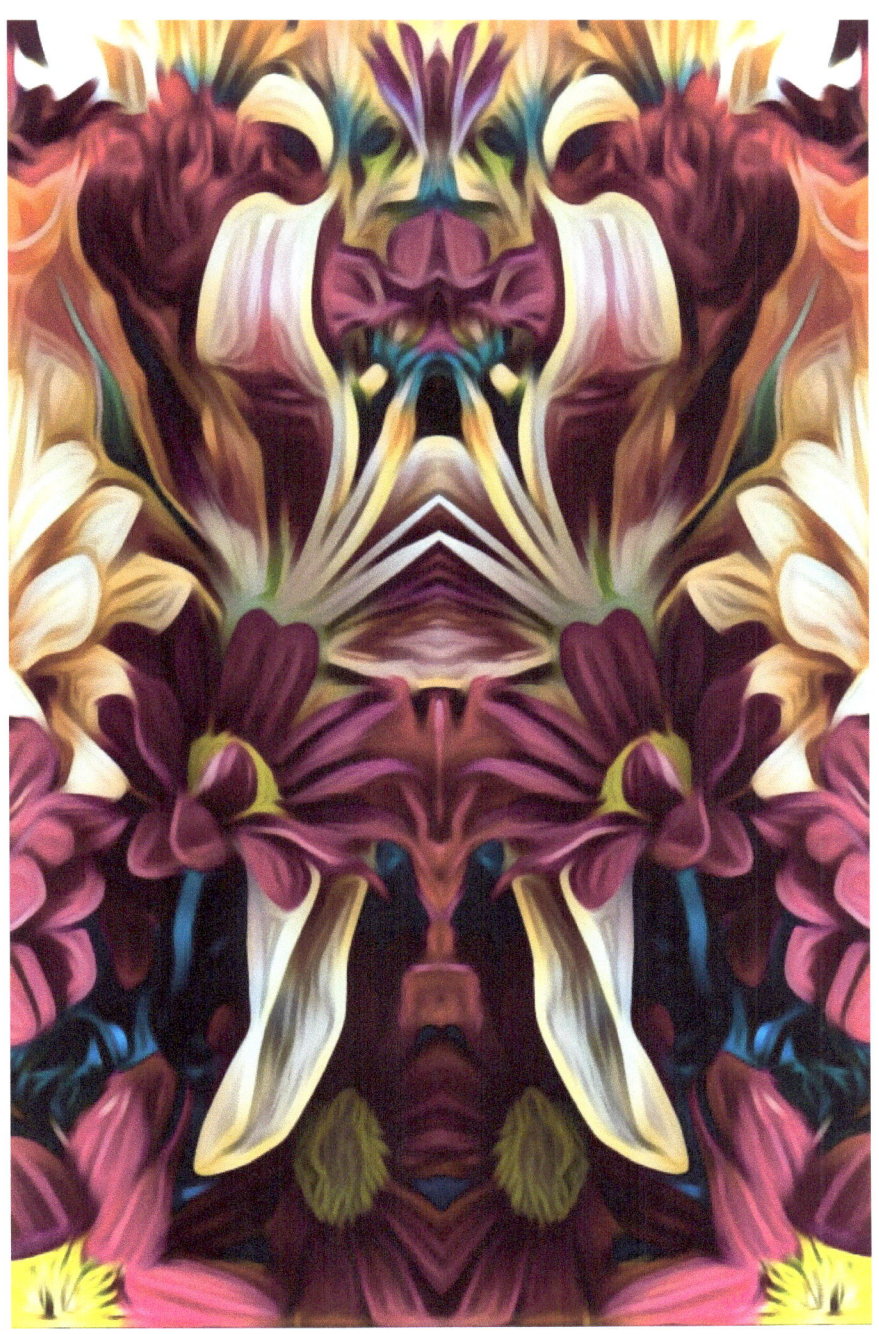

While petals suffocate in the howling of storms

Outis: A Nursing Elegy

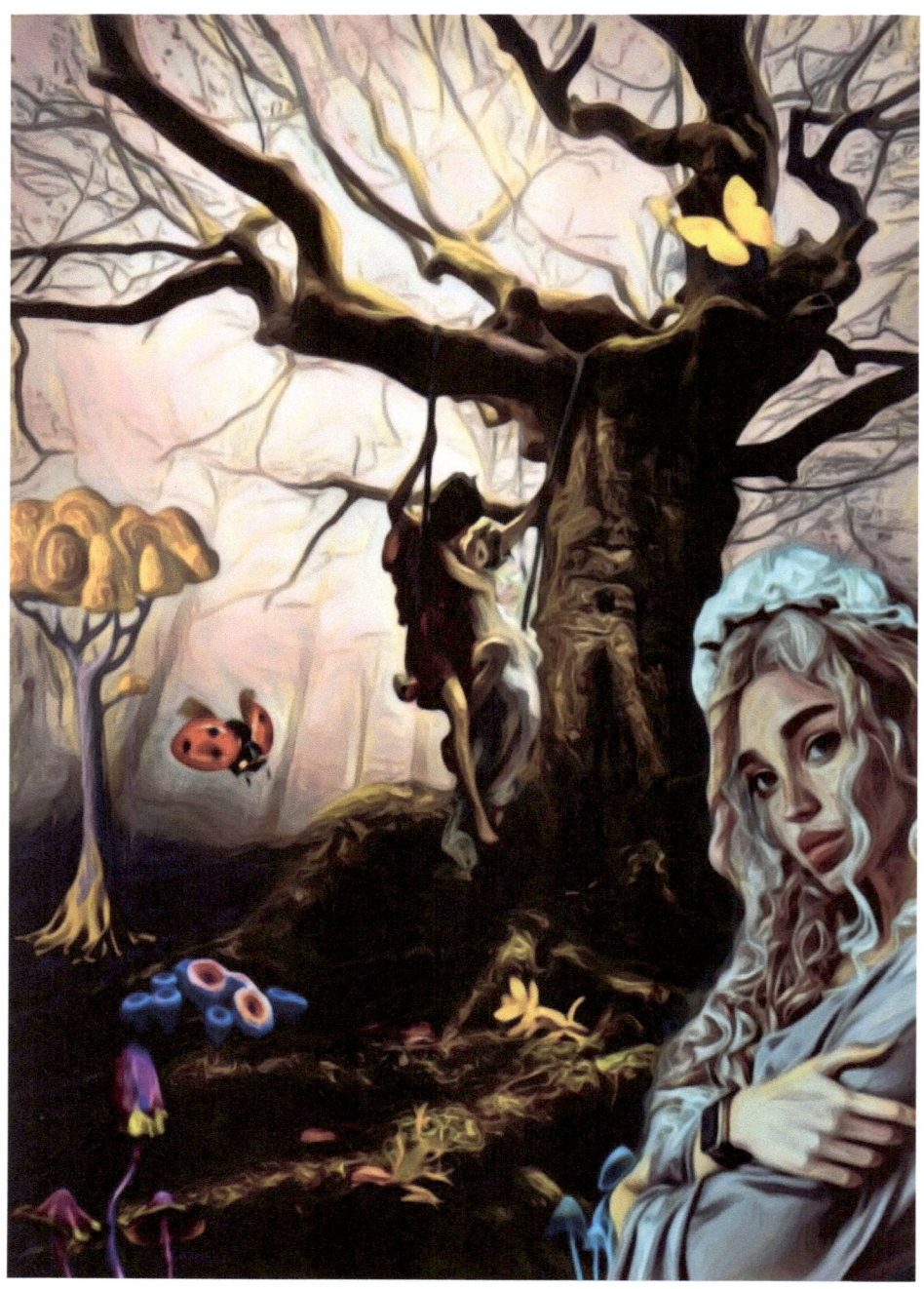

And the thorns can draw fresh blood from the plucking mourns.

Outis: A Nursing Elegy

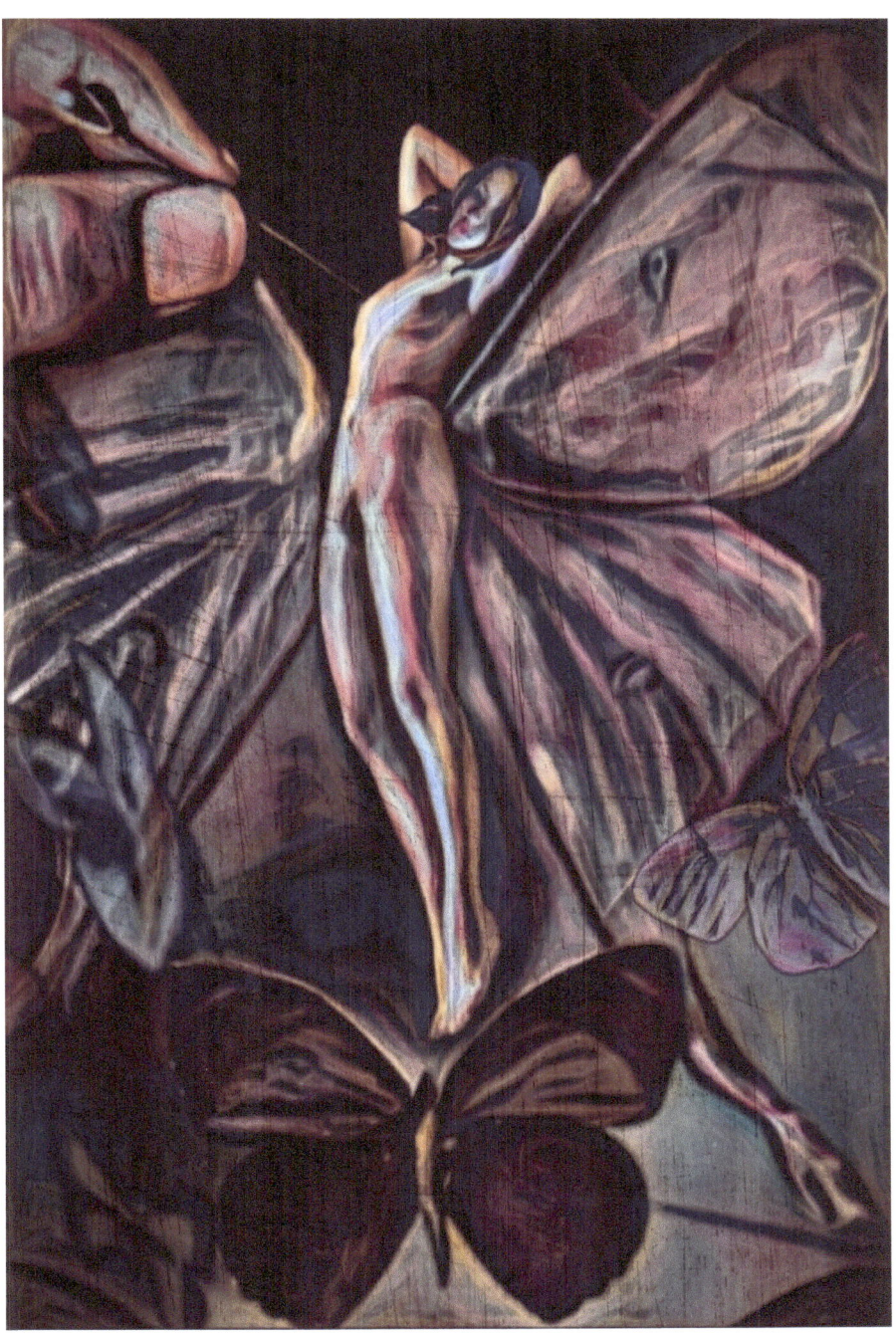

The lilacs, in full bloom, cut short for grief's display:

Outis: A Nursing Elegy

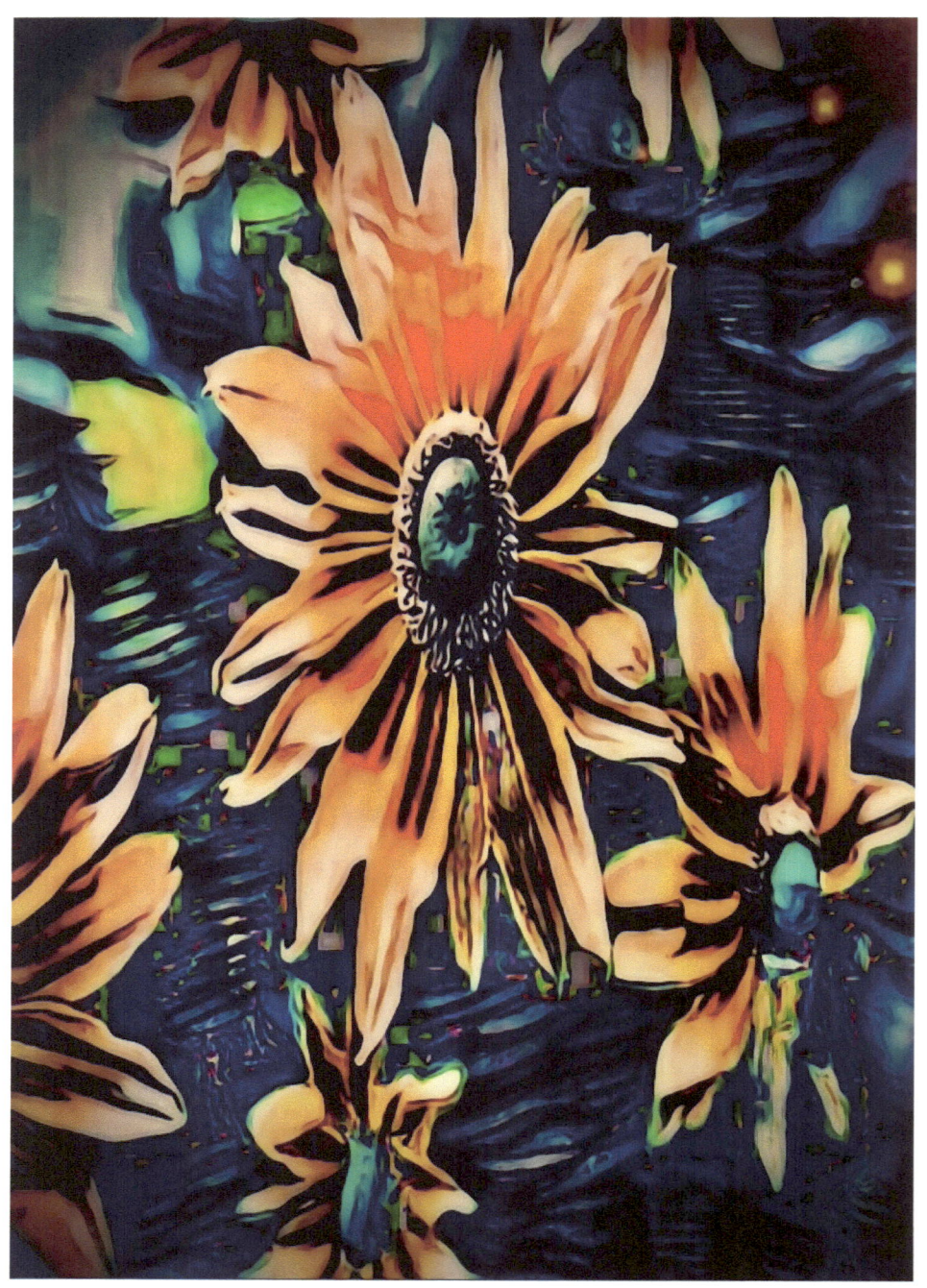

A symbol that's seen but not always understood;

Outis: A Nursing Elegy

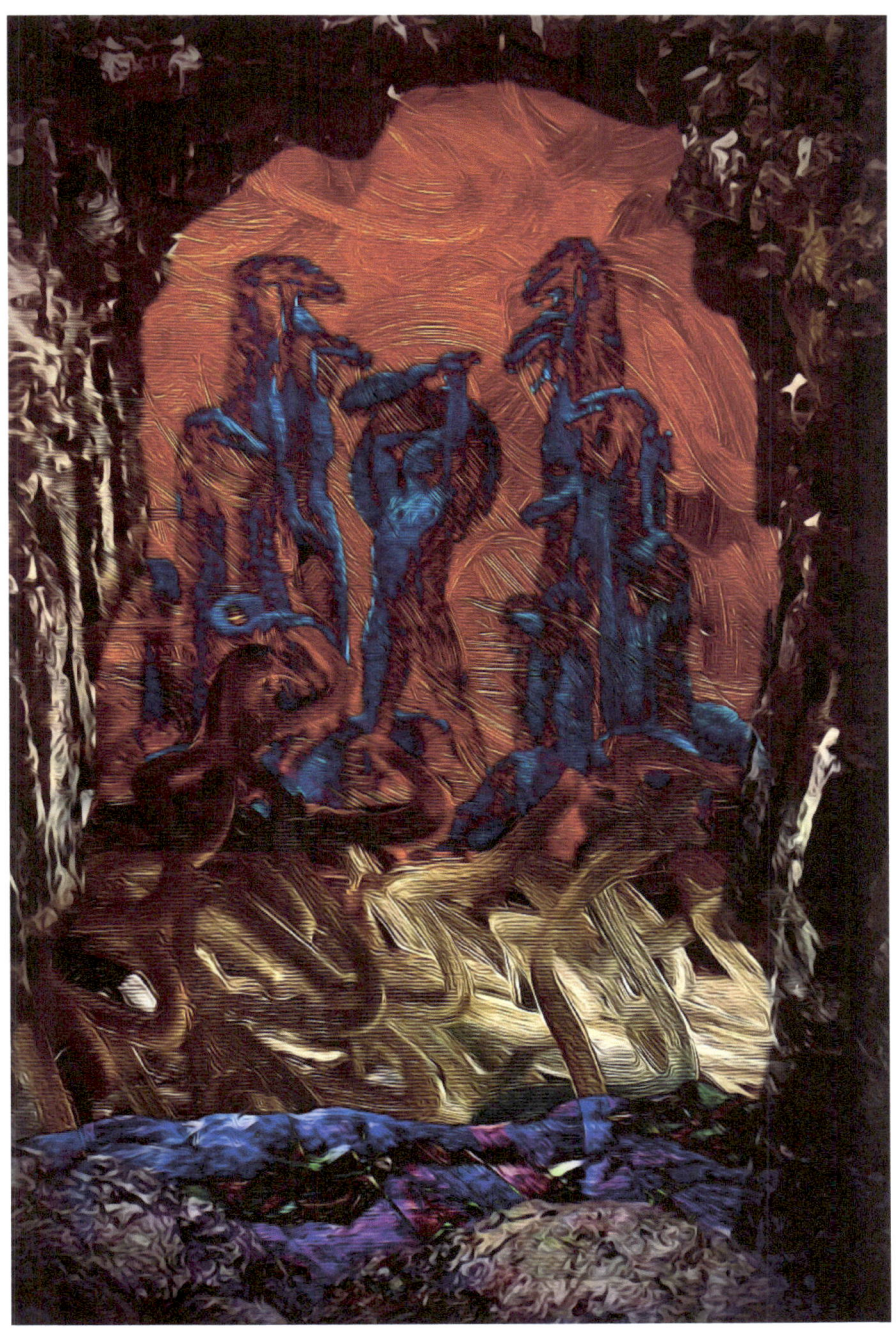

The perennial destined to return someday,

Outis: A Nursing Elegy

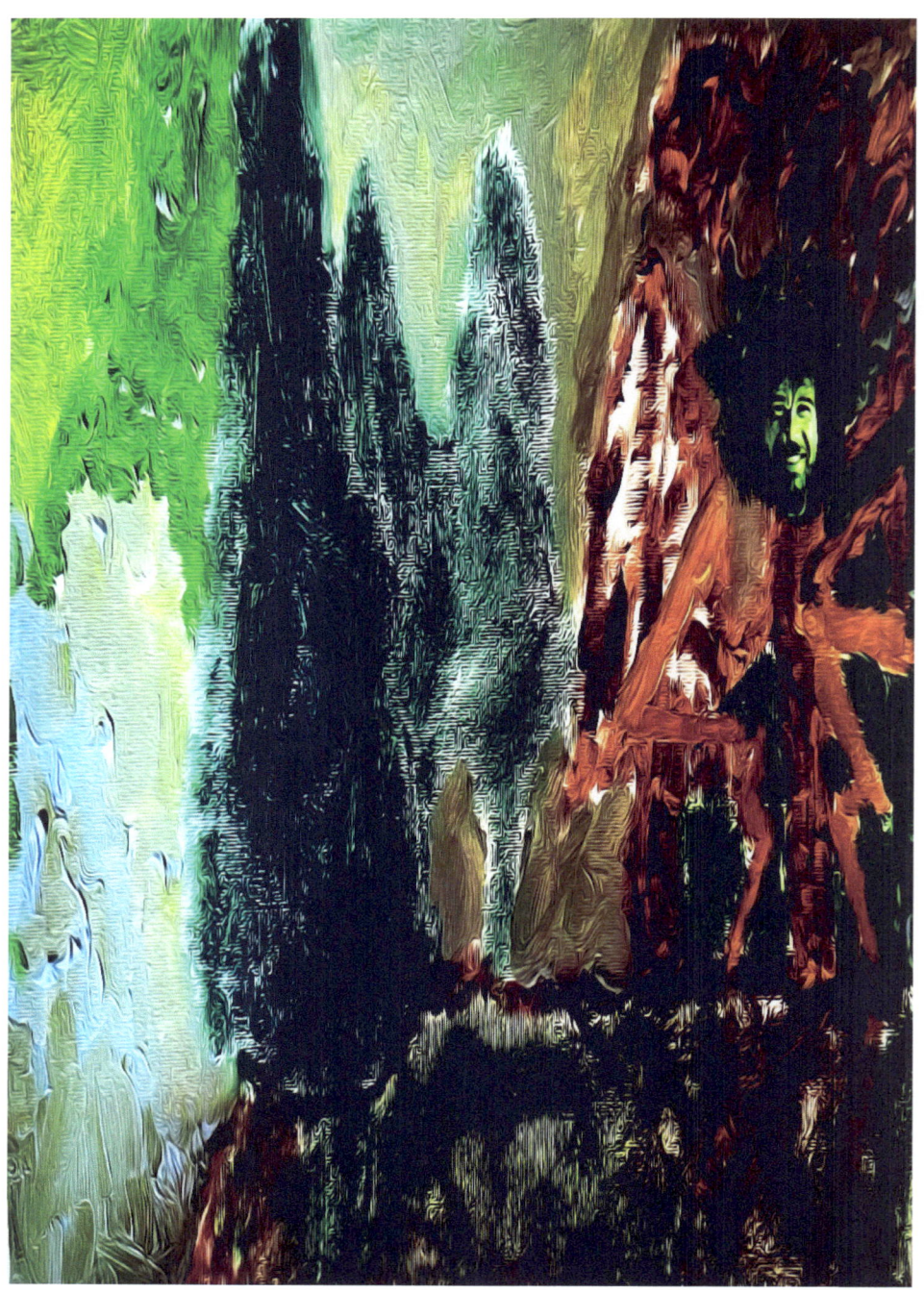

Not as the resurrection of flower and stem

Outis: A Nursing Elegy

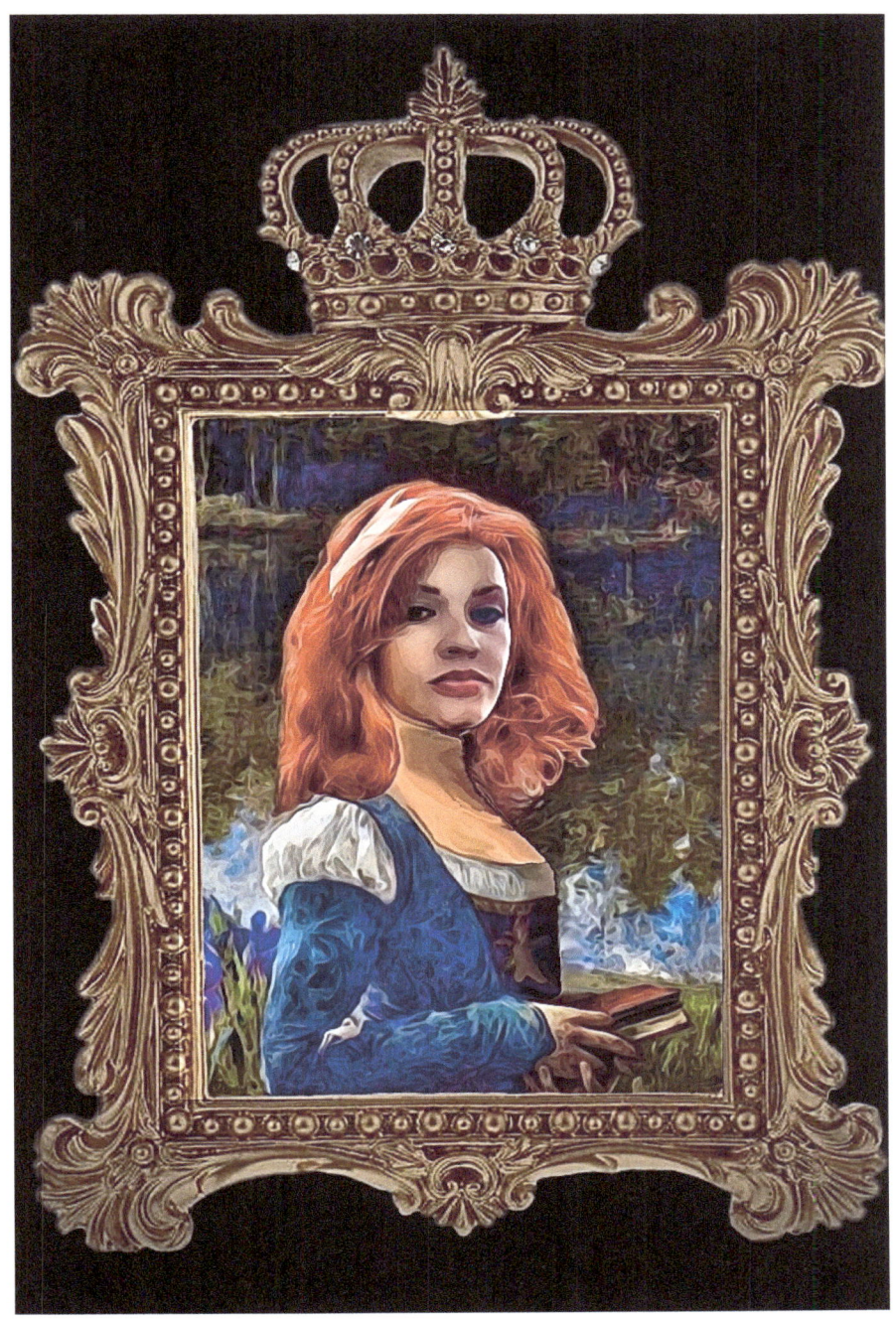

But as the legacy of a root that withstood

Outis: A Nursing Elegy

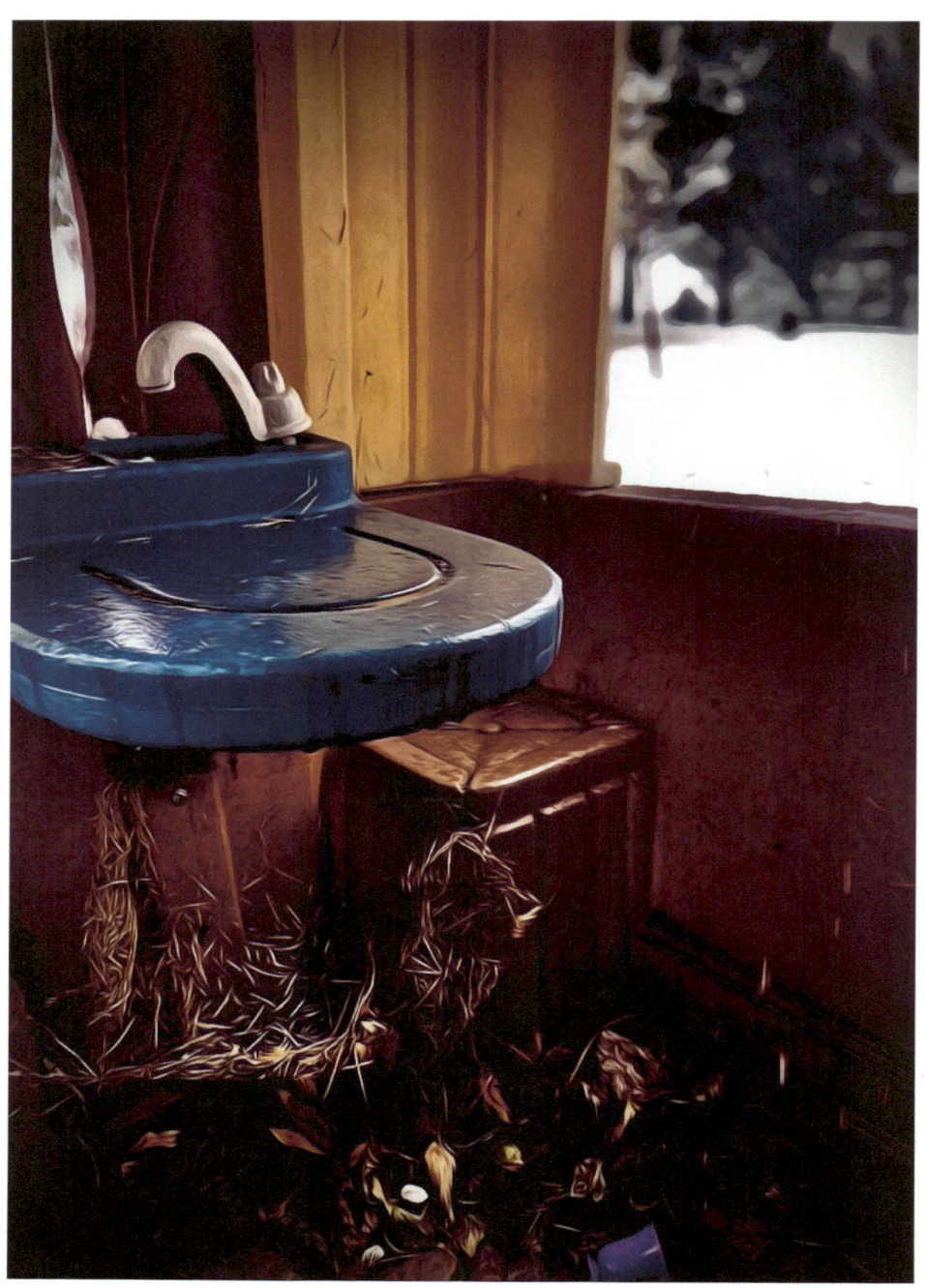

Frozen enrapture of a December condemn.

Outis: A Nursing Elegy

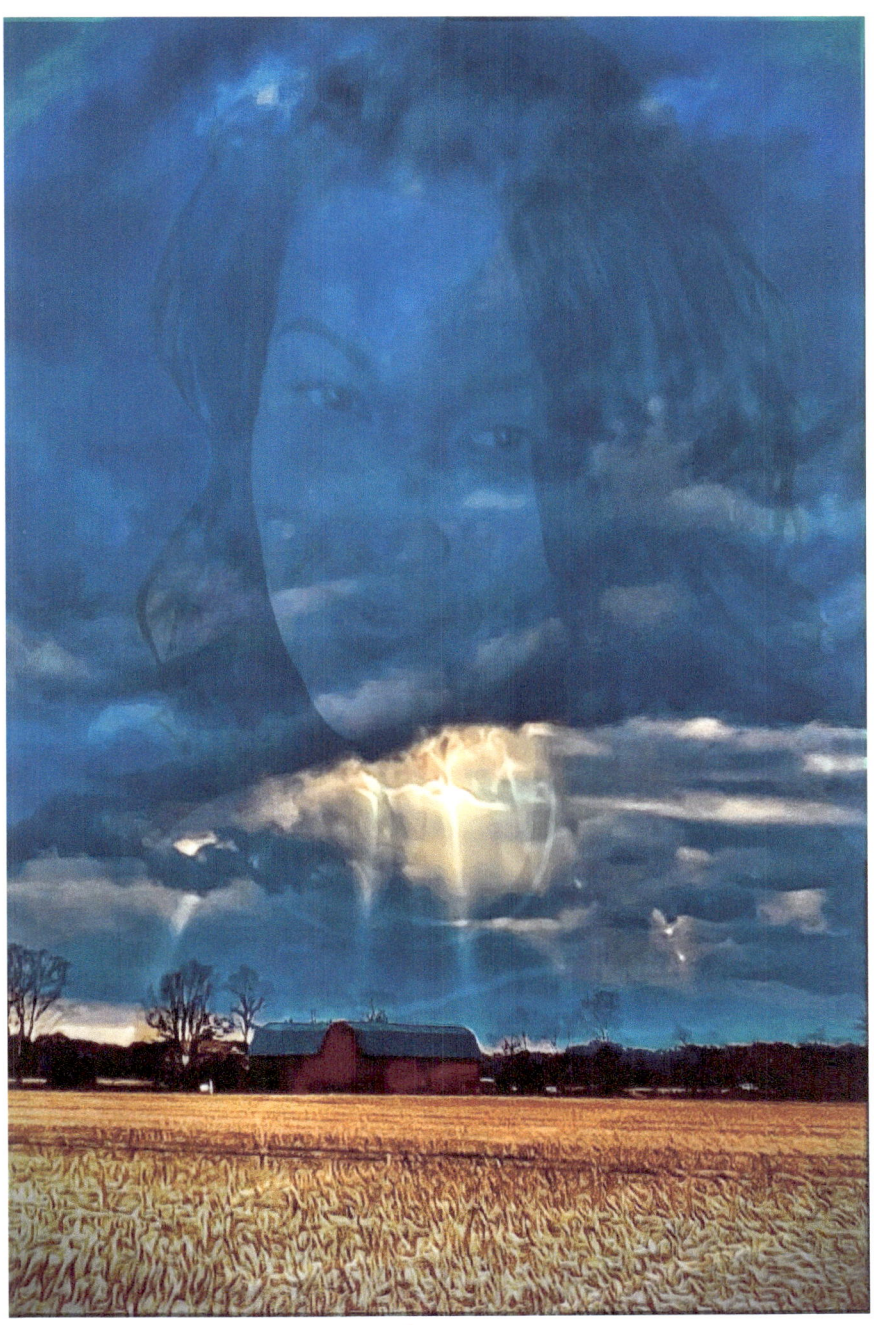

True death comes not in the reap to those who see prime;

Outis: A Nursing Elegy

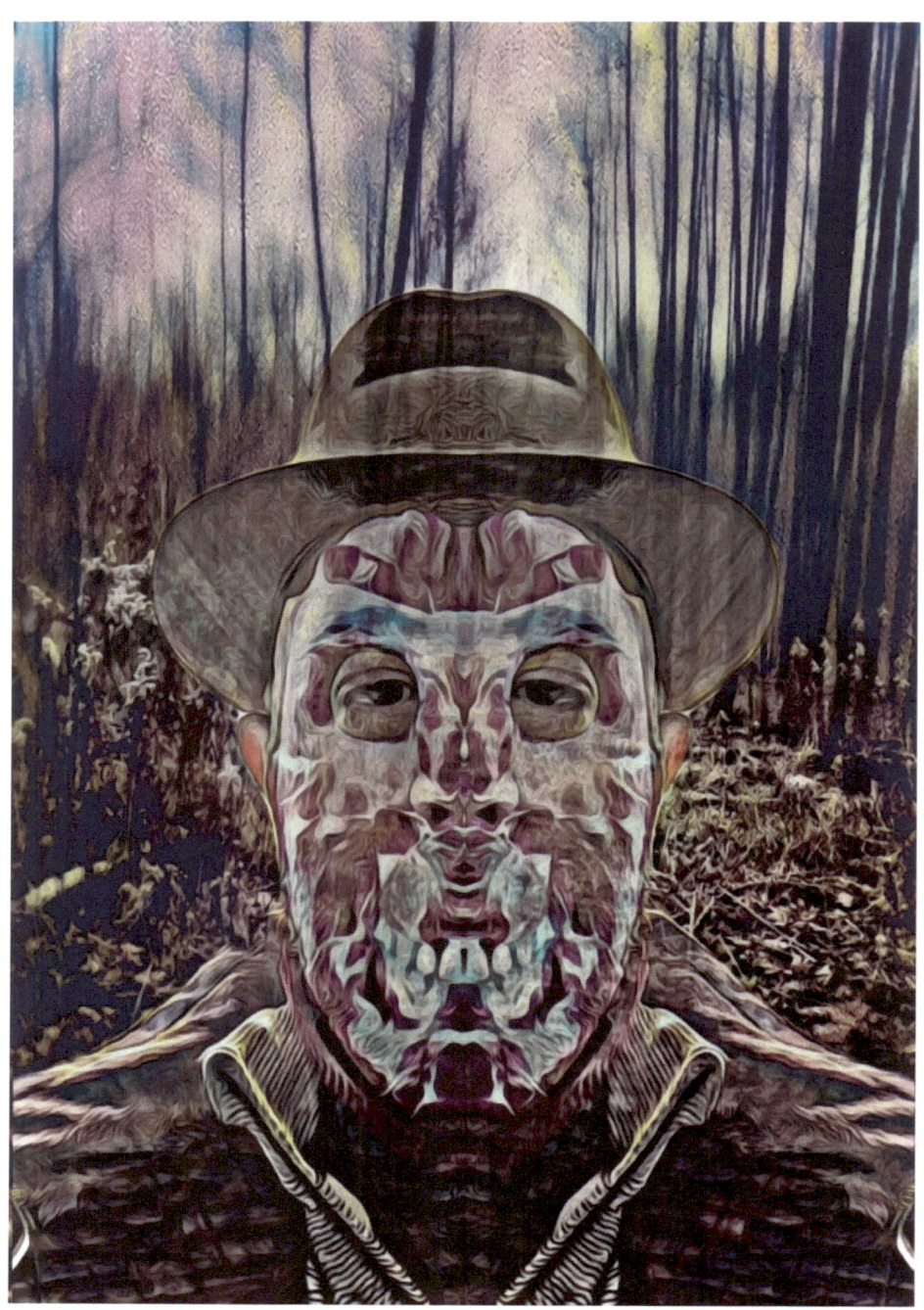

It is when decay settles upon the blossoms

Outis: A Nursing Elegy

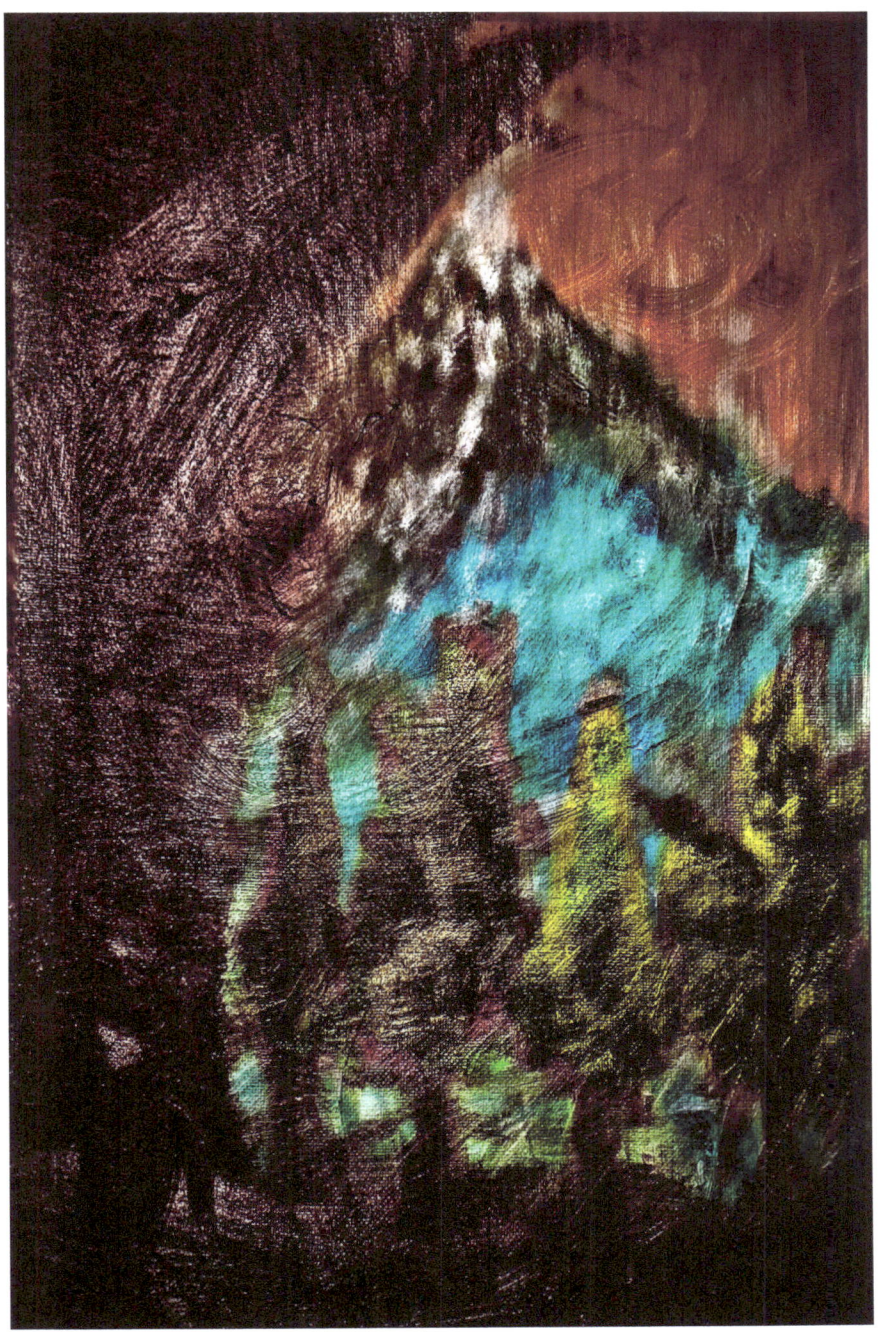

That is when the passing becomes noted in time.

Outis: A Nursing Elegy

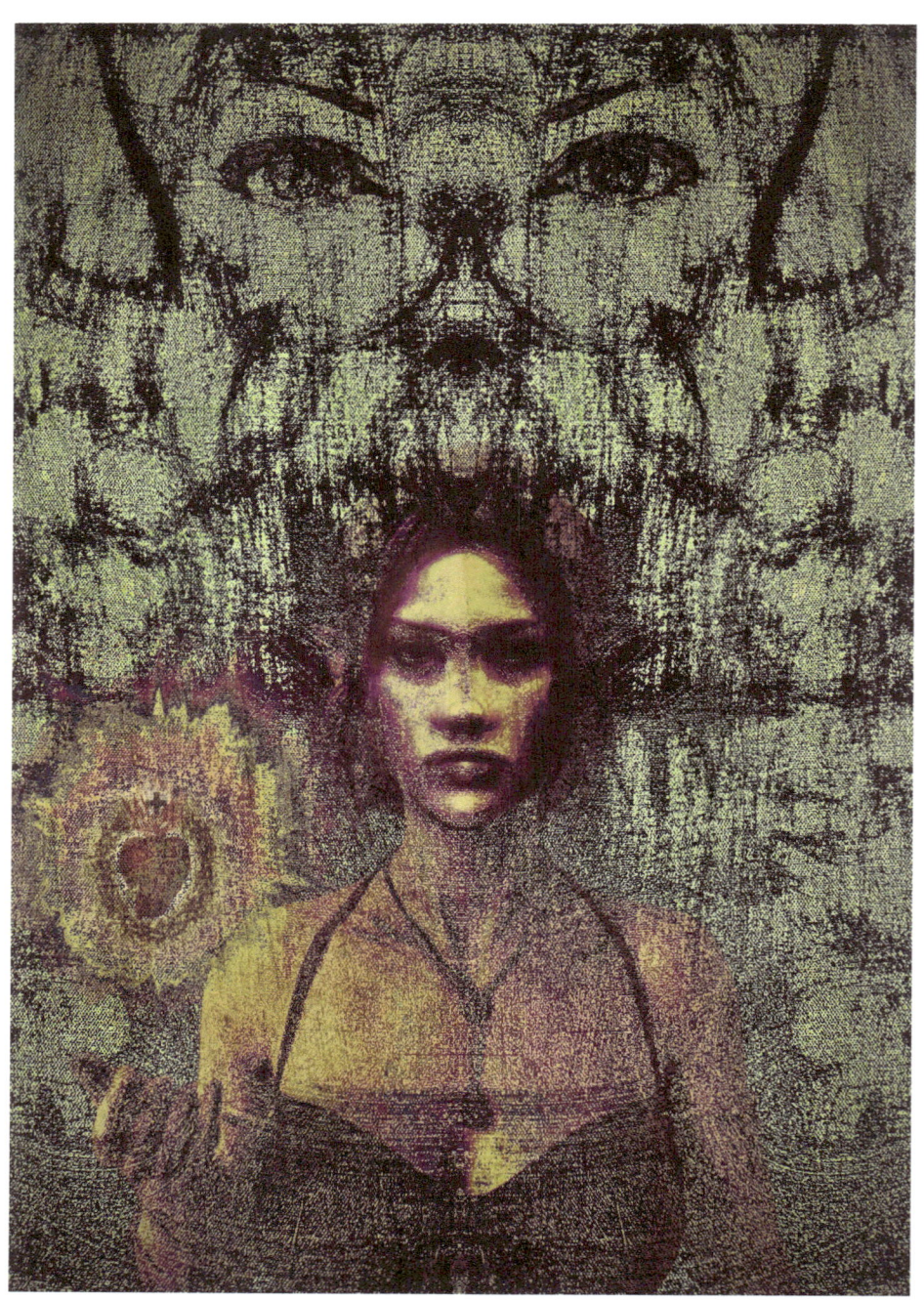

To lovers of essence, the presence lingers on

Outis: A Nursing Elegy

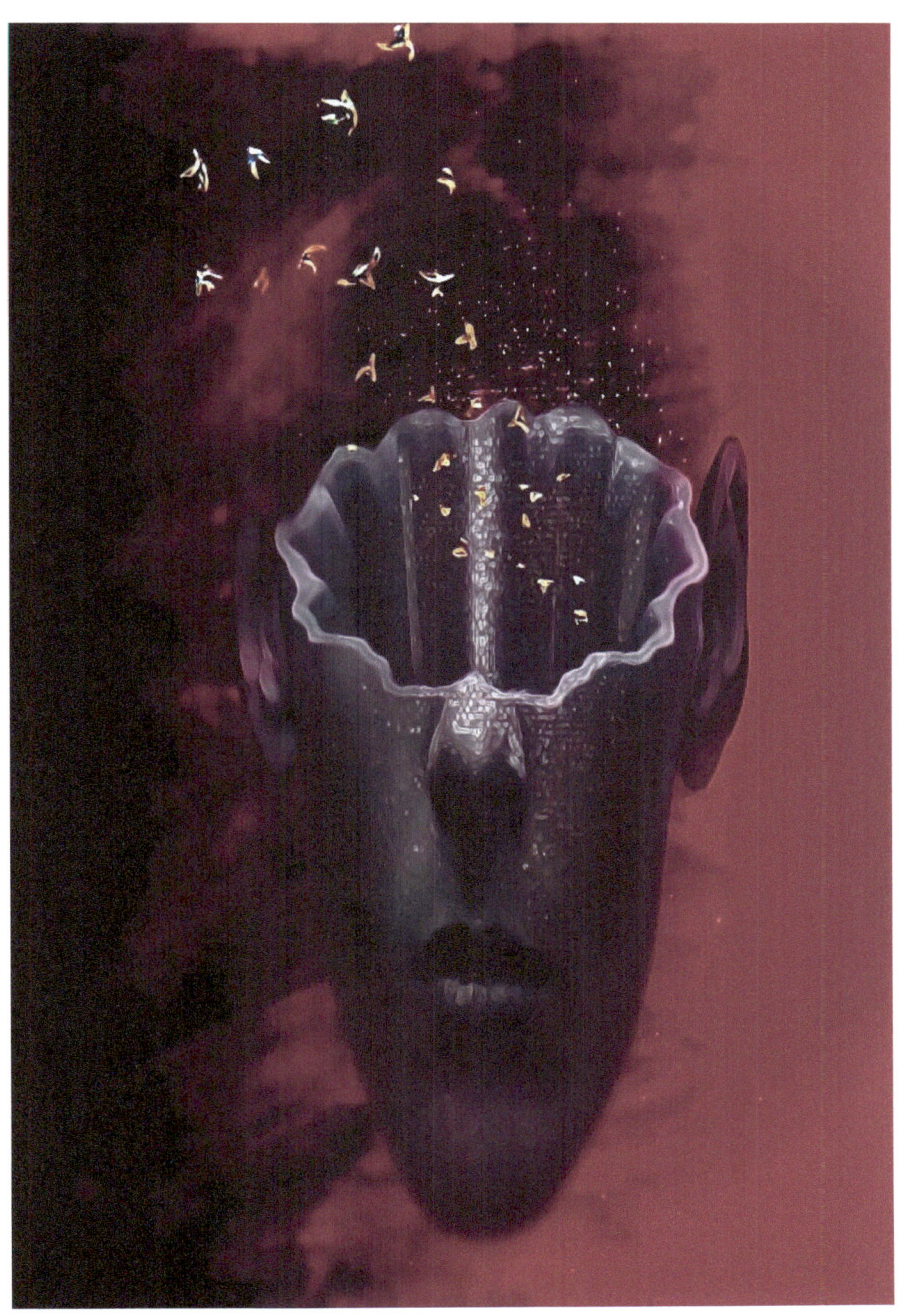

Like the soft echoing trills of woodland oscines;

Outis: A Nursing Elegy

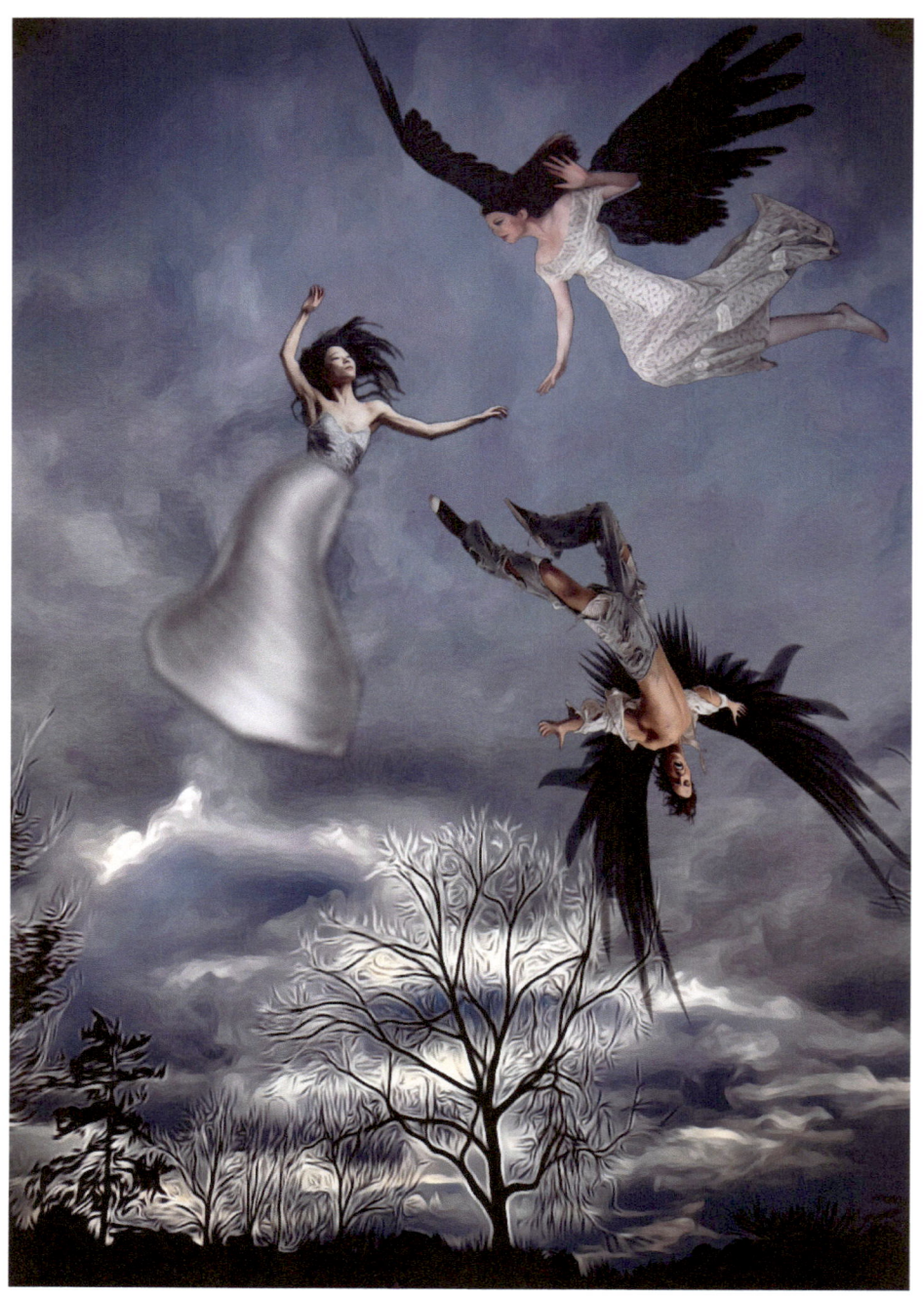

Life lives on in life, even when todays are gone,

Outis: A Nursing Elegy

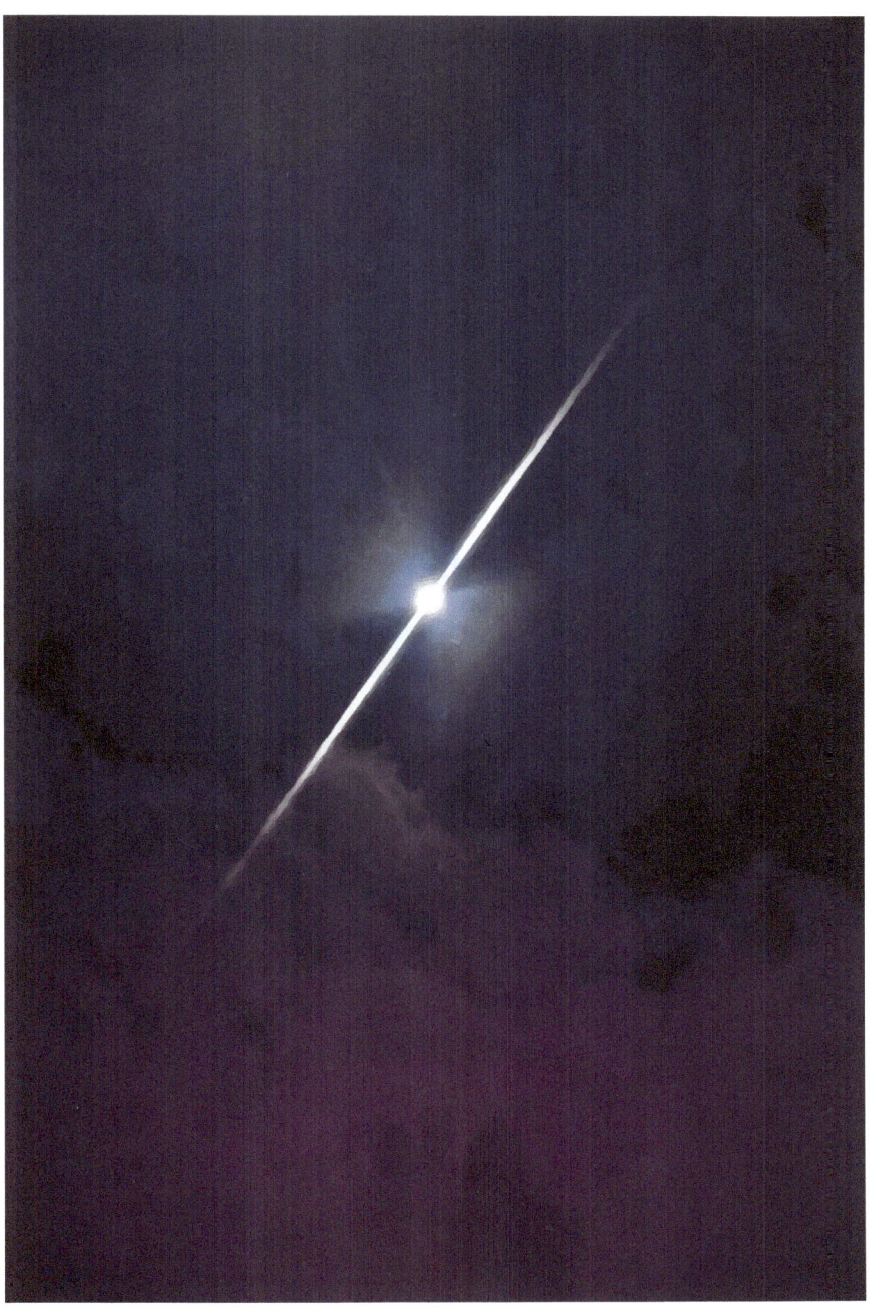

To be the lightning flash, not the thunder after:

Outis: A Nursing Elegy

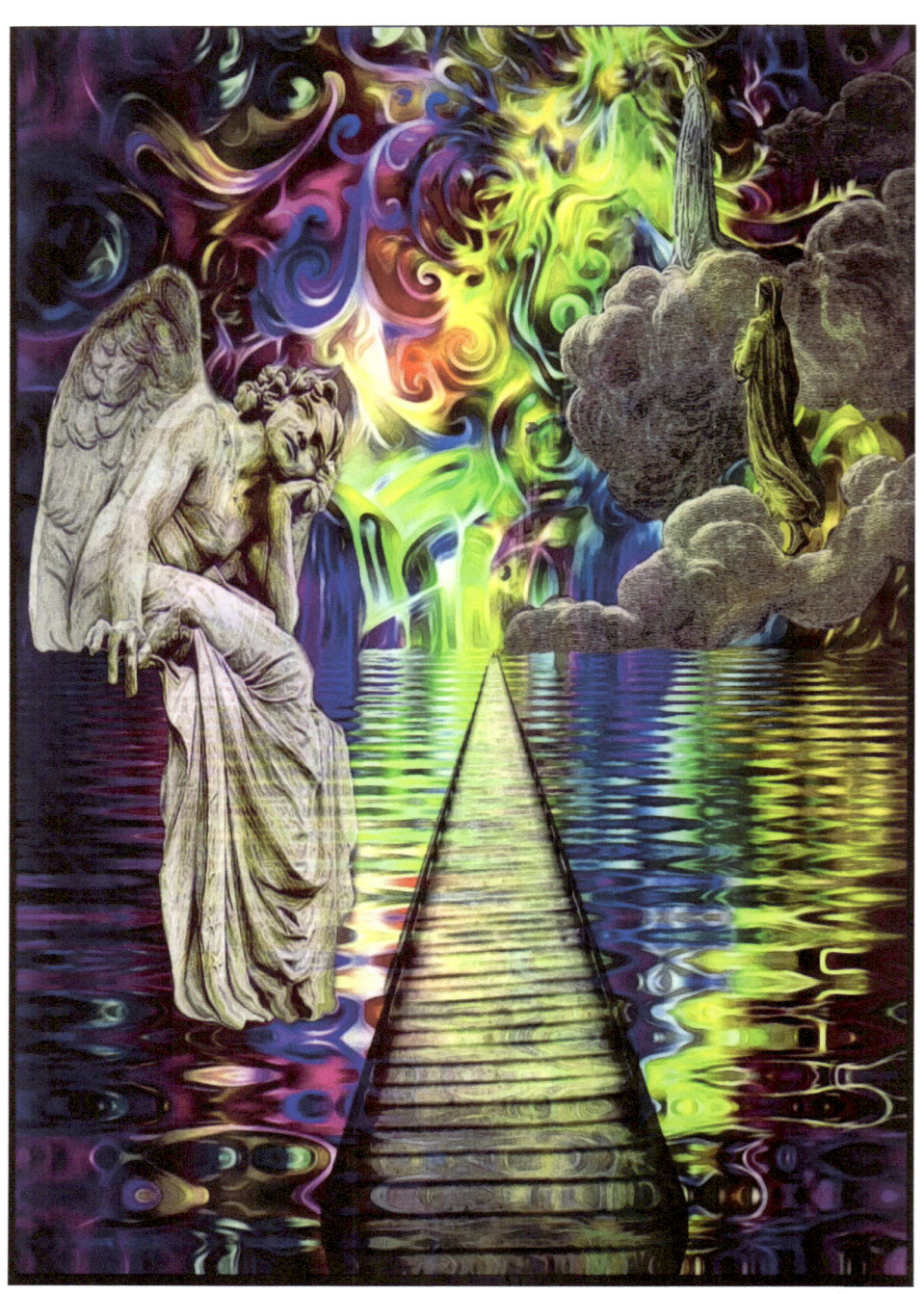

The eternity now, mortality later.

Outis: A Nursing Elegy

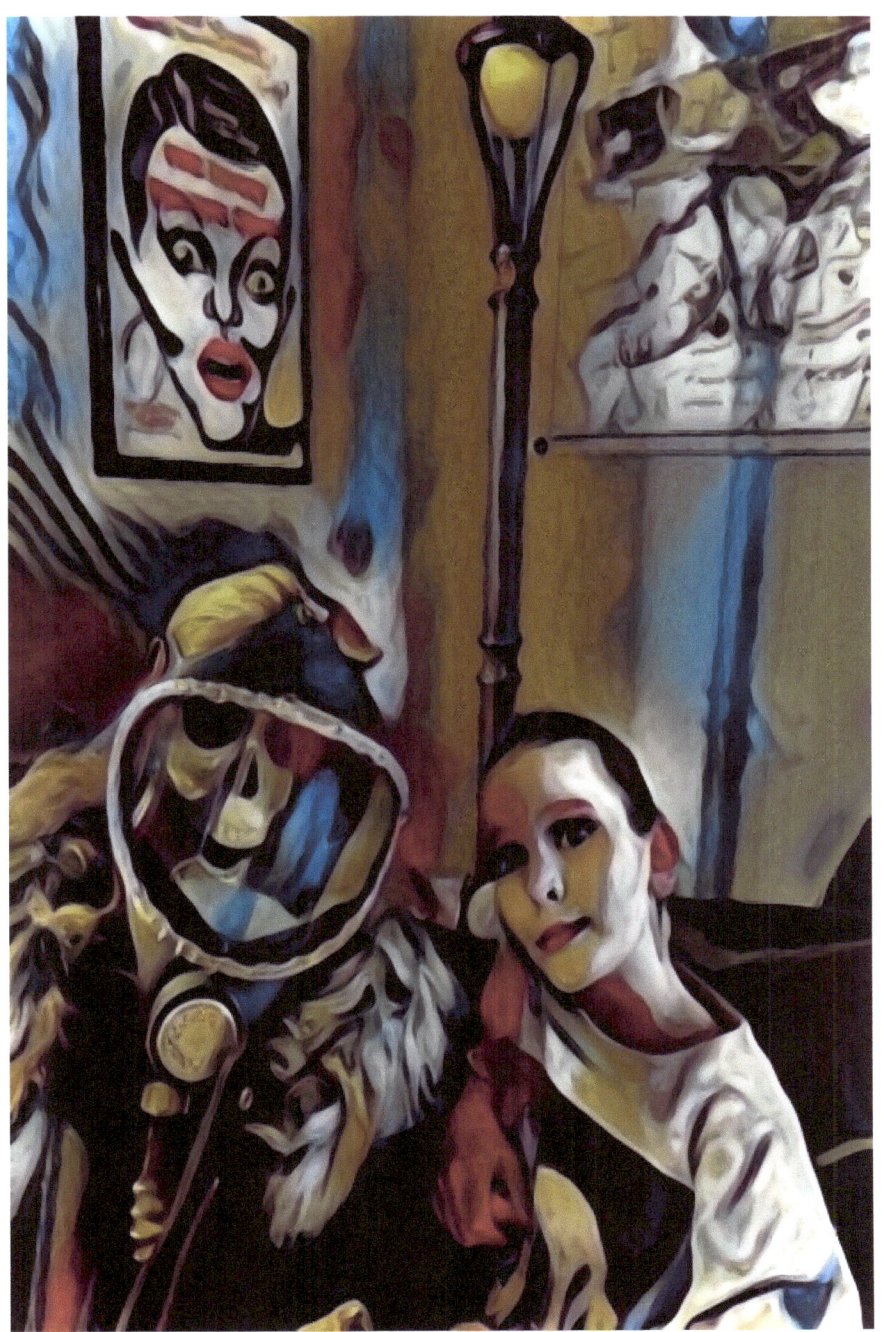

Born to a fate of death,

Outis: A Nursing Elegy

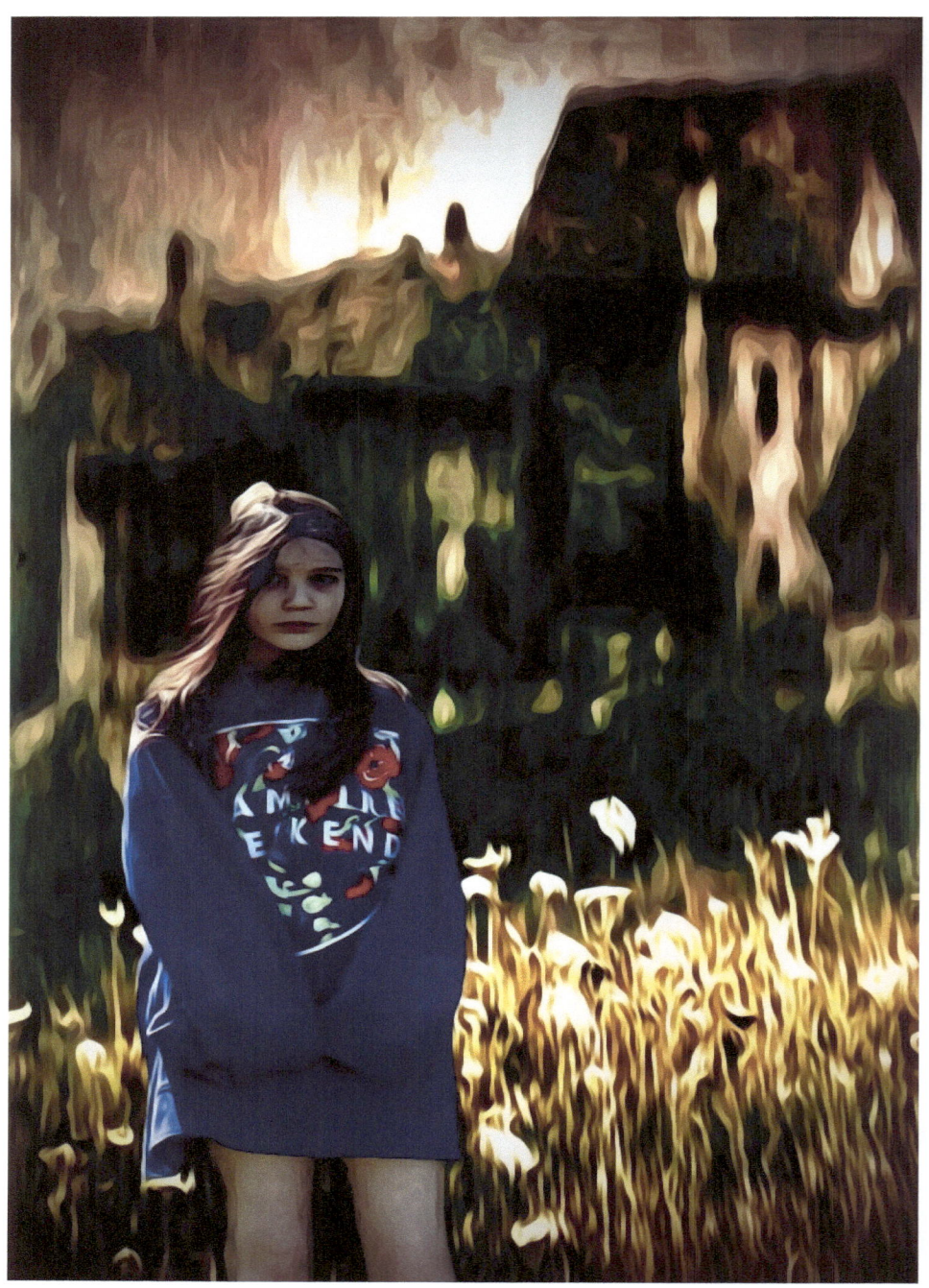

Life follows scripts of chance.

Outis: A Nursing Elegy

Cruel and unfair, the world offers no place to hide.

Outis: A Nursing Elegy

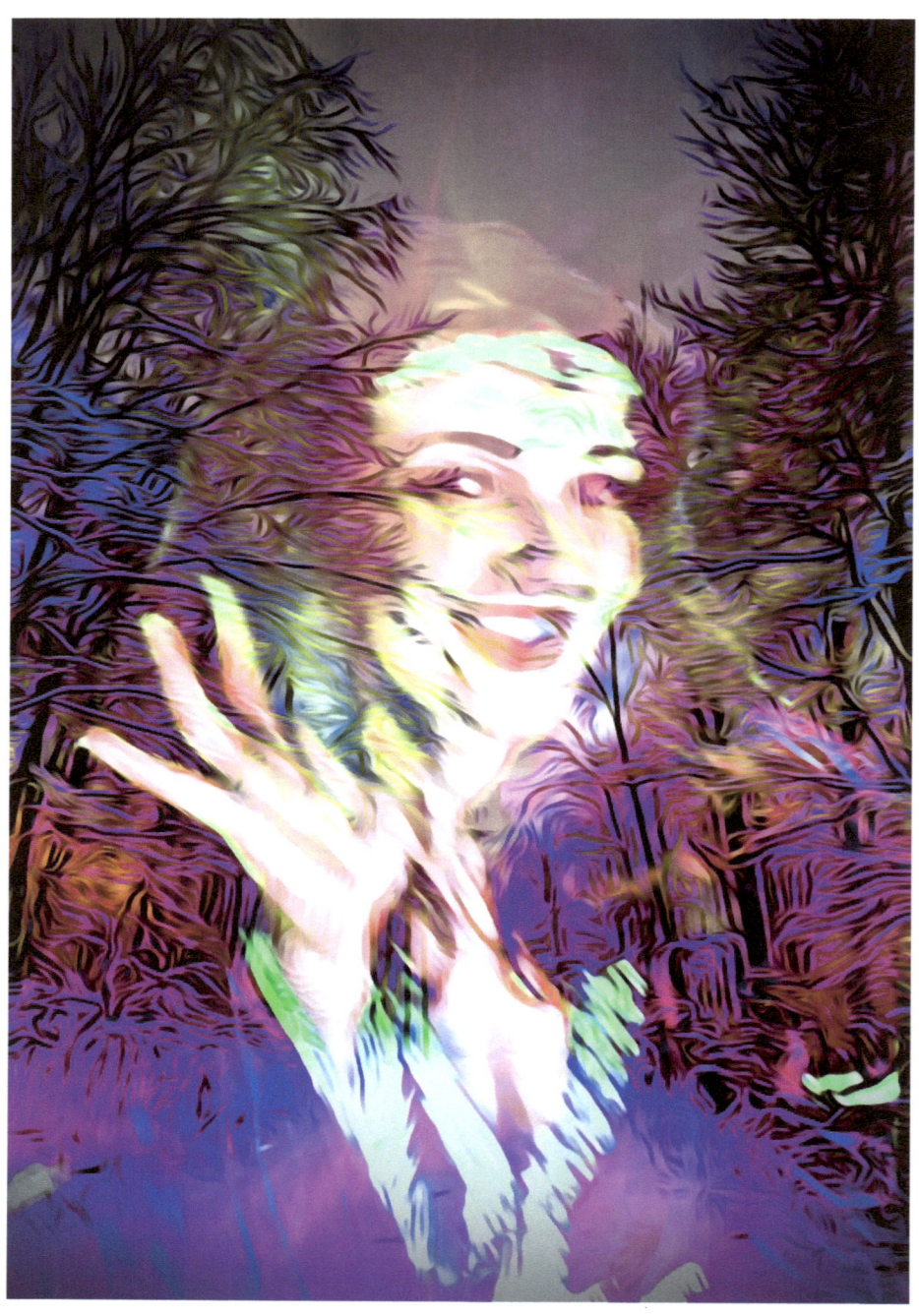

A suffering romances those that takes a stance.

Outis: A Nursing Elegy

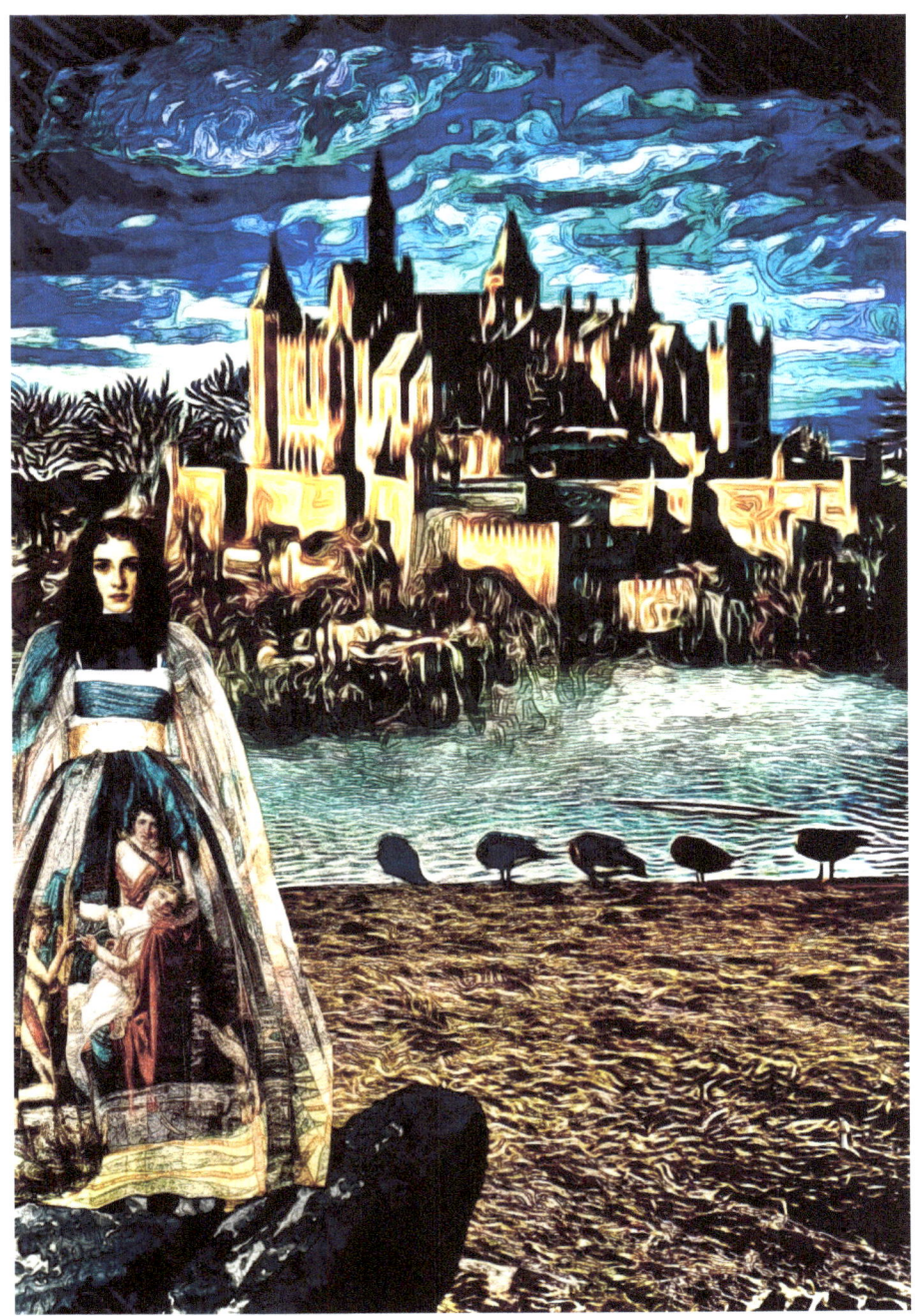

Those that aim to please earns a hollowness in time.

Outis: A Nursing Elegy

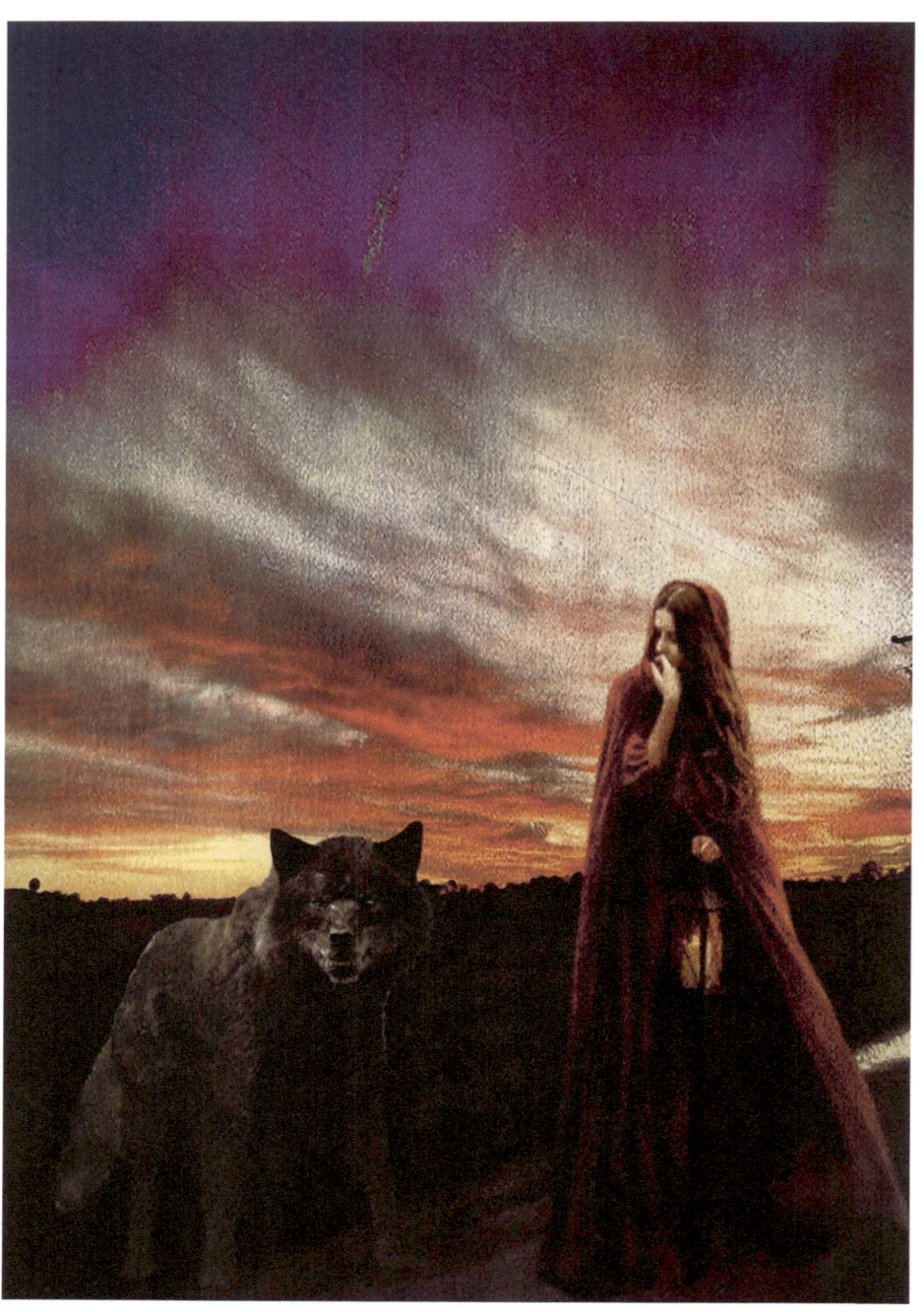

Oblivion awaits those that blacken eyes of pry.

Outis: A Nursing Elegy

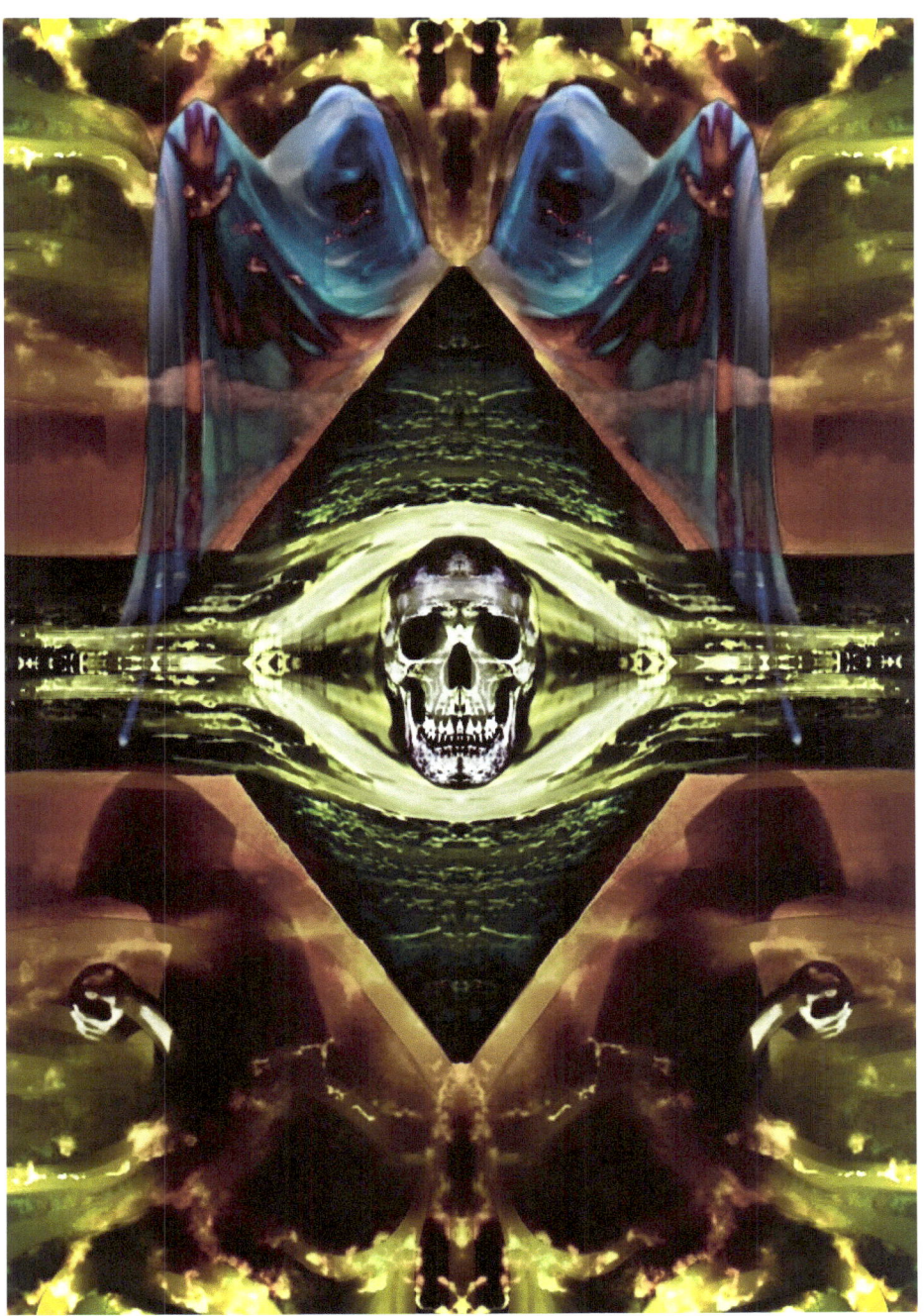

Martyr, libertine or hermit- all fall in their climb.

Outis: A Nursing Elegy

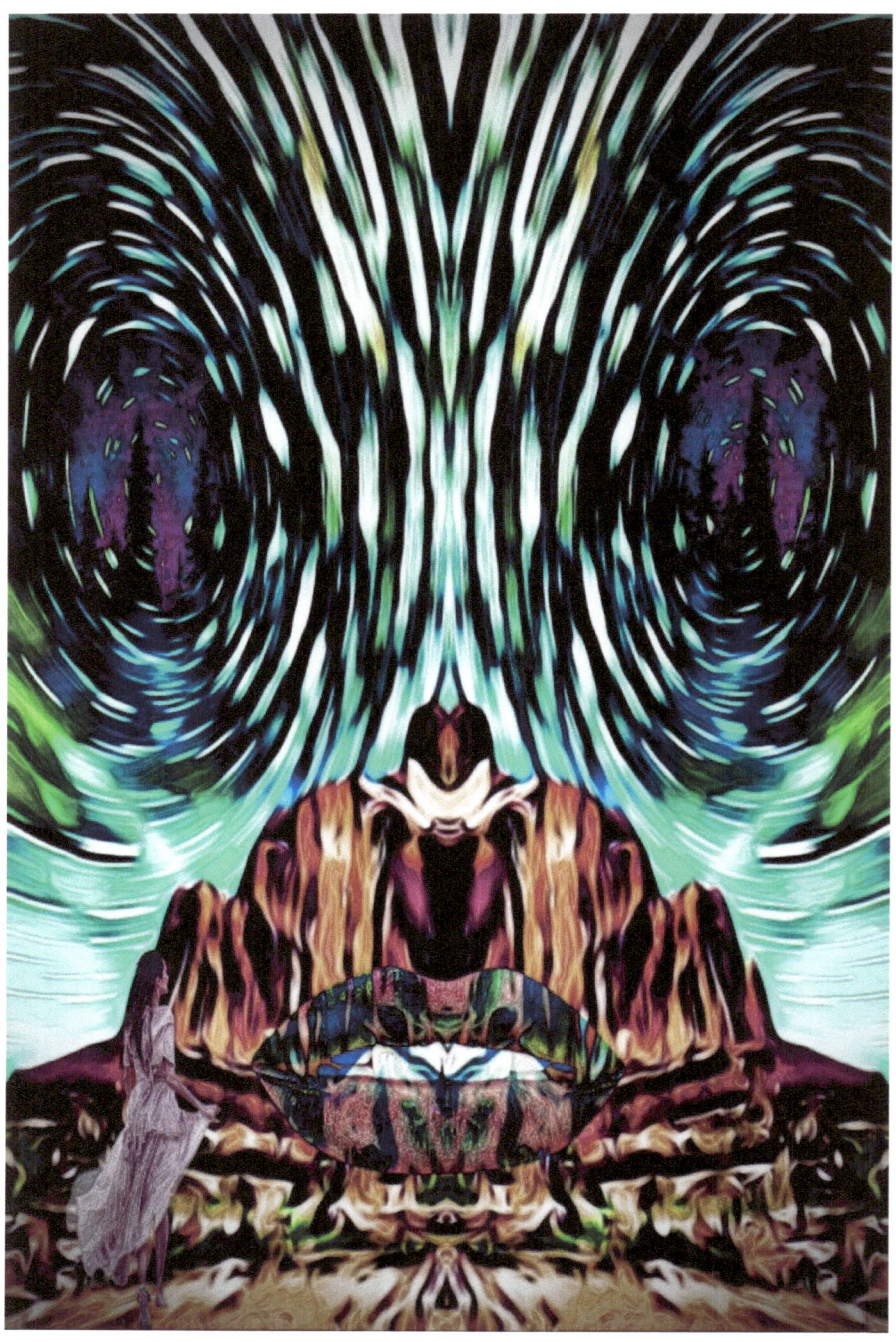

Fame is like breath- known today, forgotten tomorrow.

Outis: A Nursing Elegy

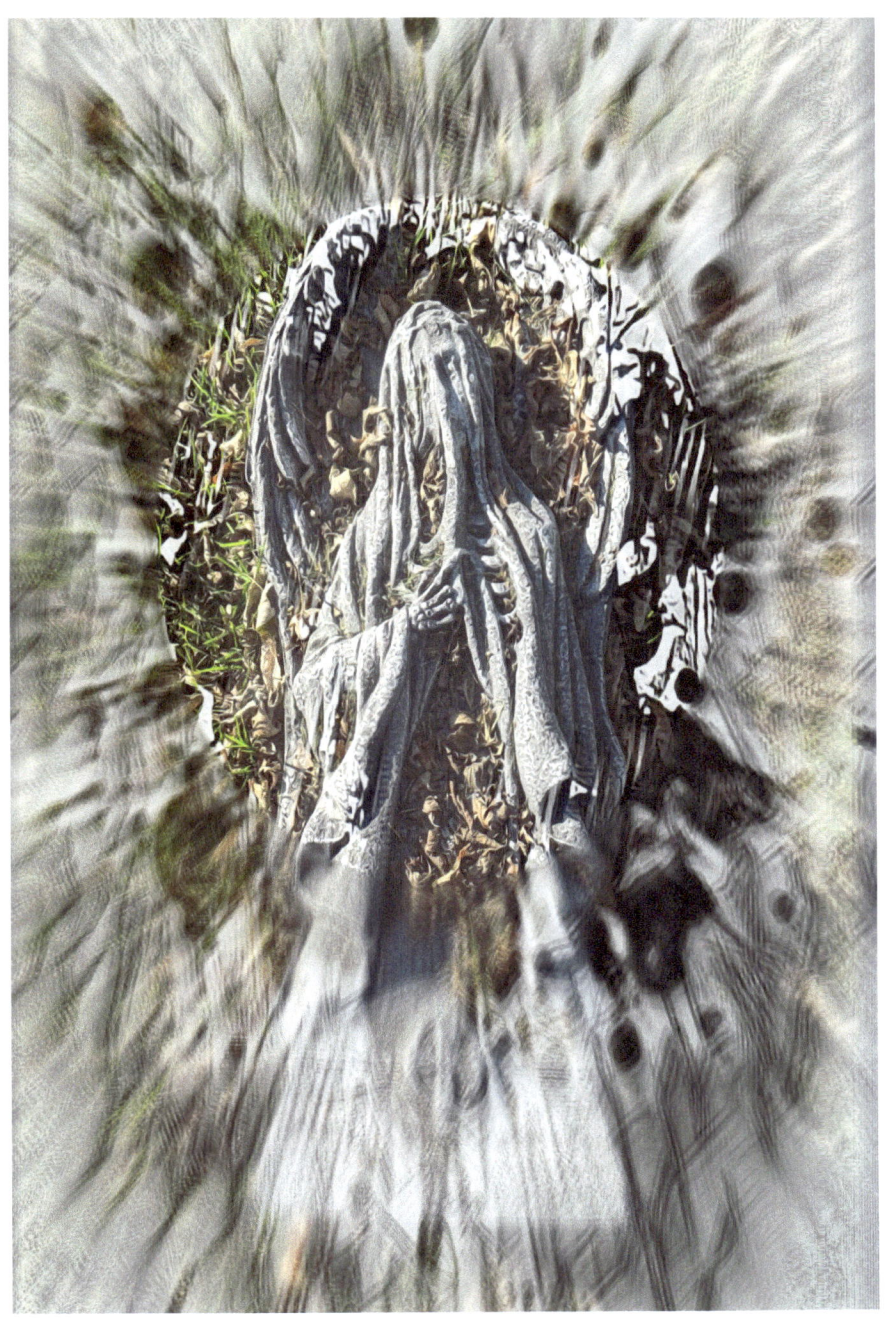

Rows of withered gravestones,

Outis: A Nursing Elegy

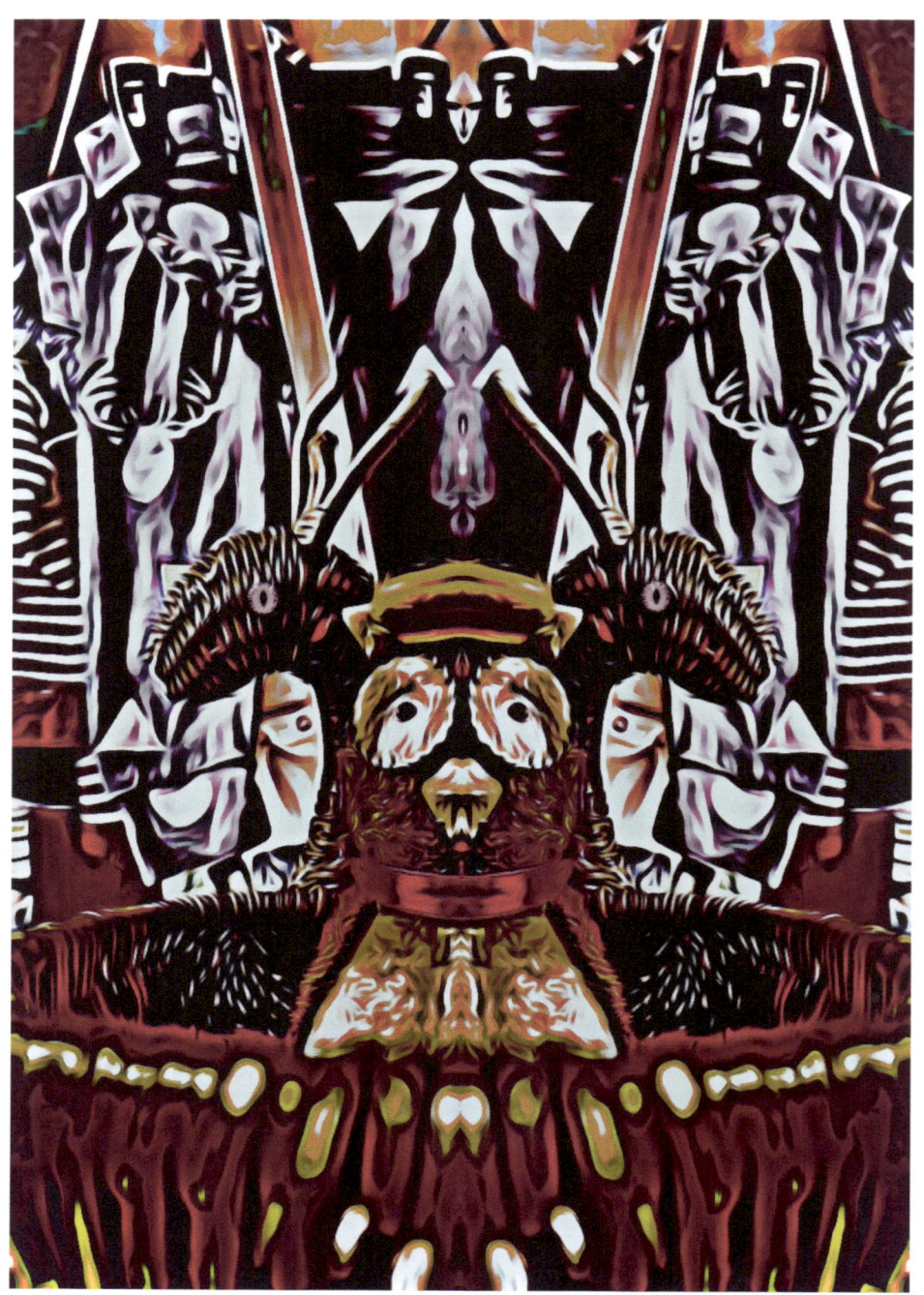

Markers for rotten bones:

Outis: A Nursing Elegy

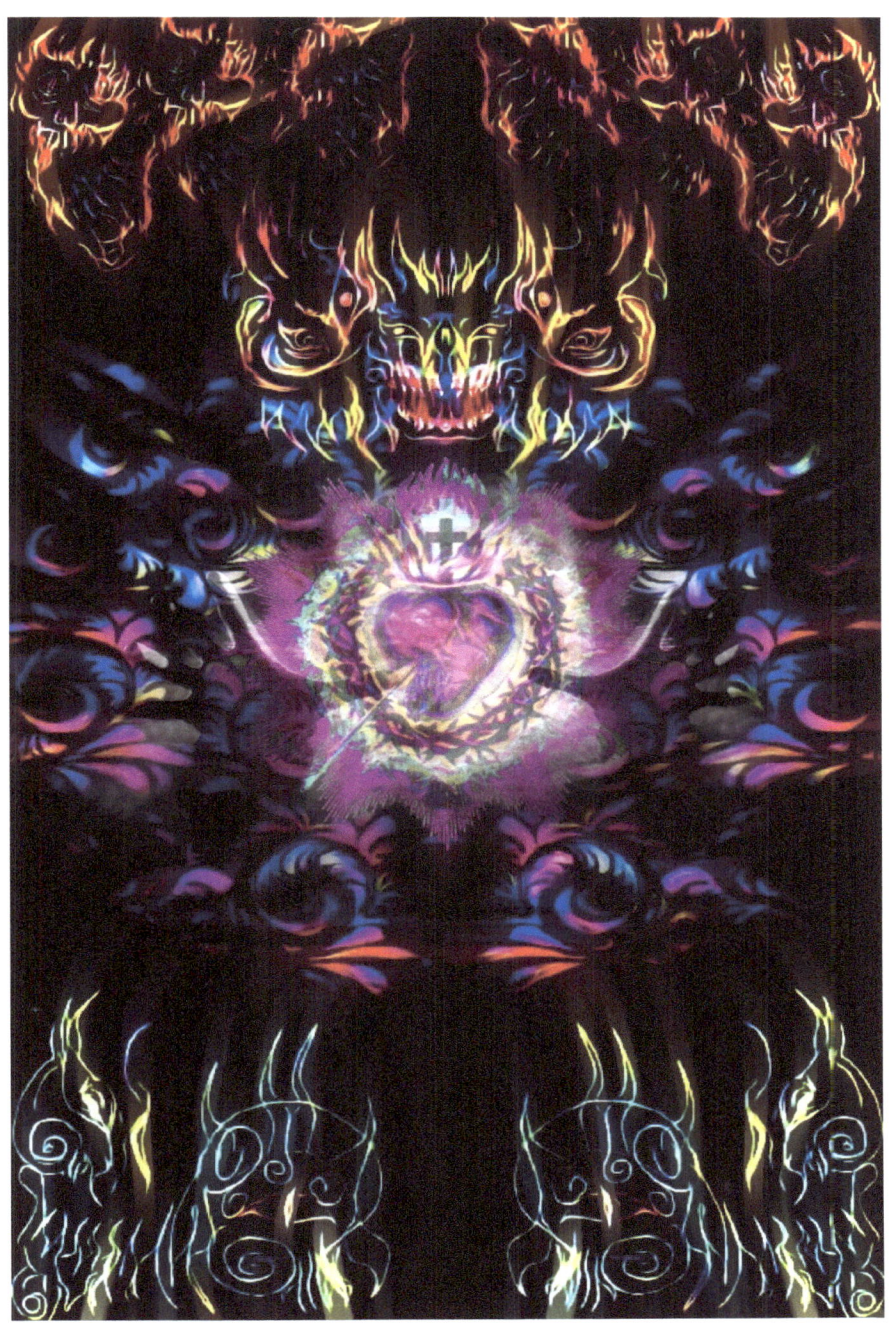

Testaments of purpose,

Outis: A Nursing Elegy

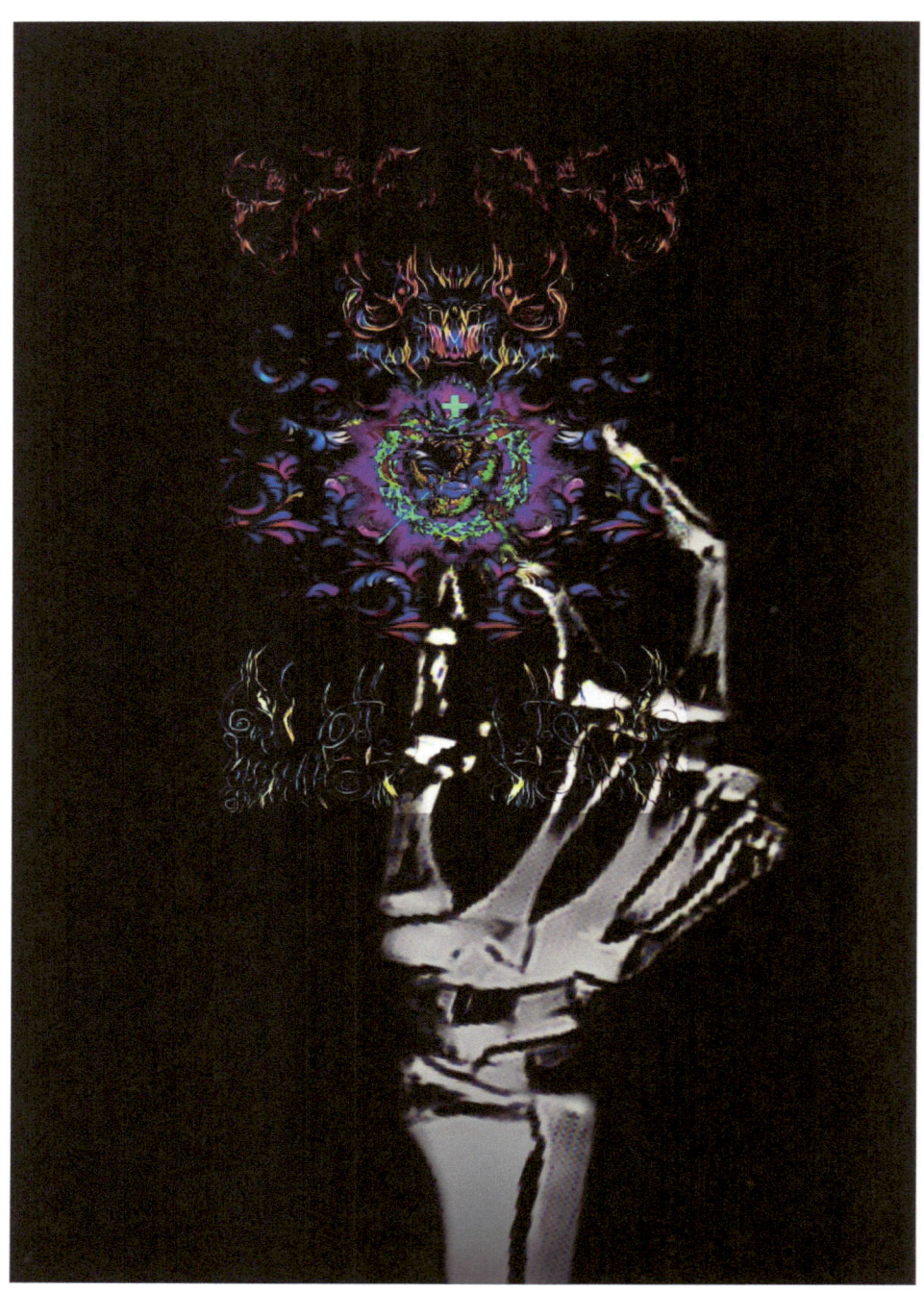

Memories of sorrow.

Outis: A Nursing Elegy

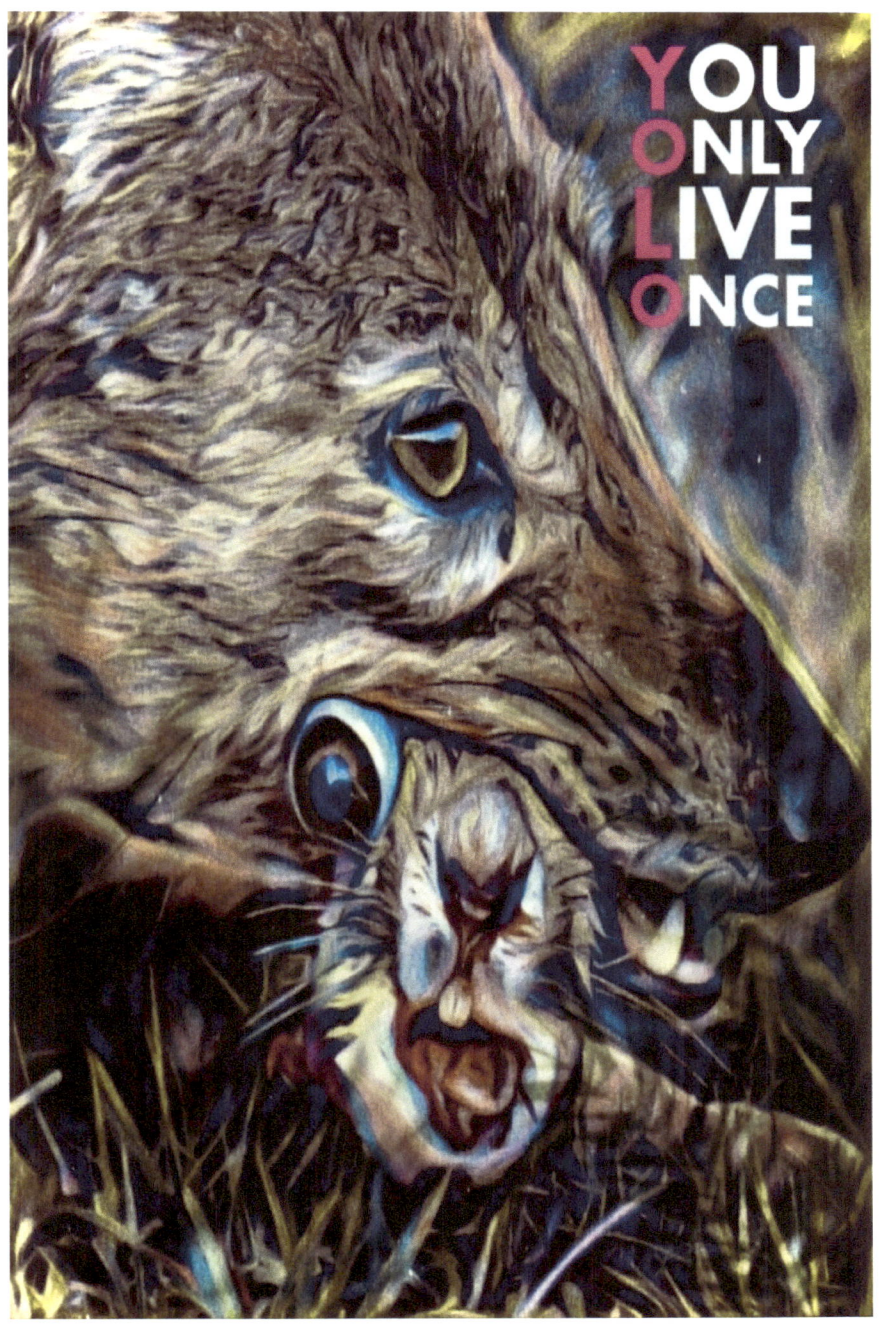

How the-dead-once-lived continues to throb in bloodstreams

Outis: A Nursing Elegy

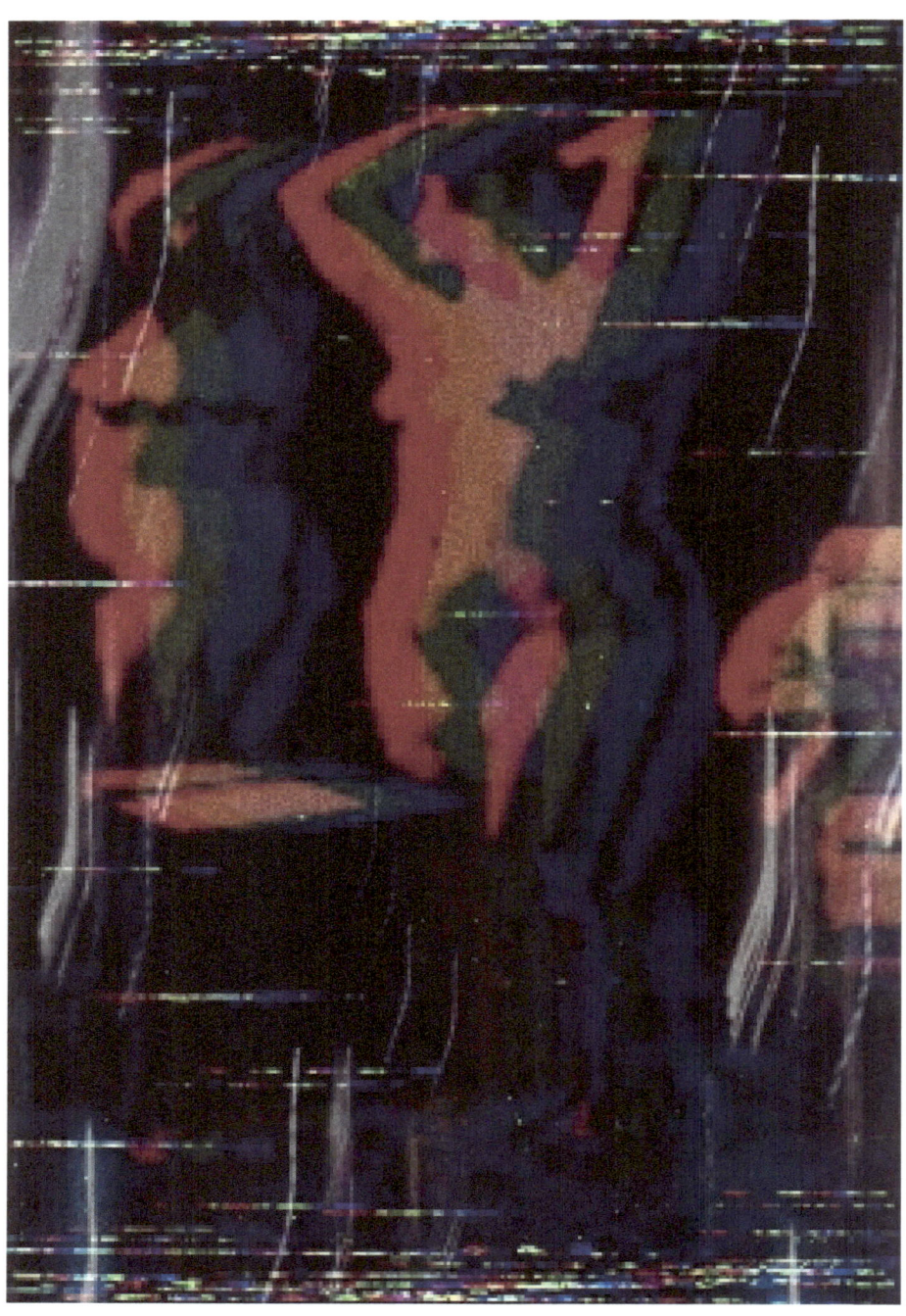

As ghosts of rhythm, the architects of hormones. . .

Outis: A Nursing Elegy

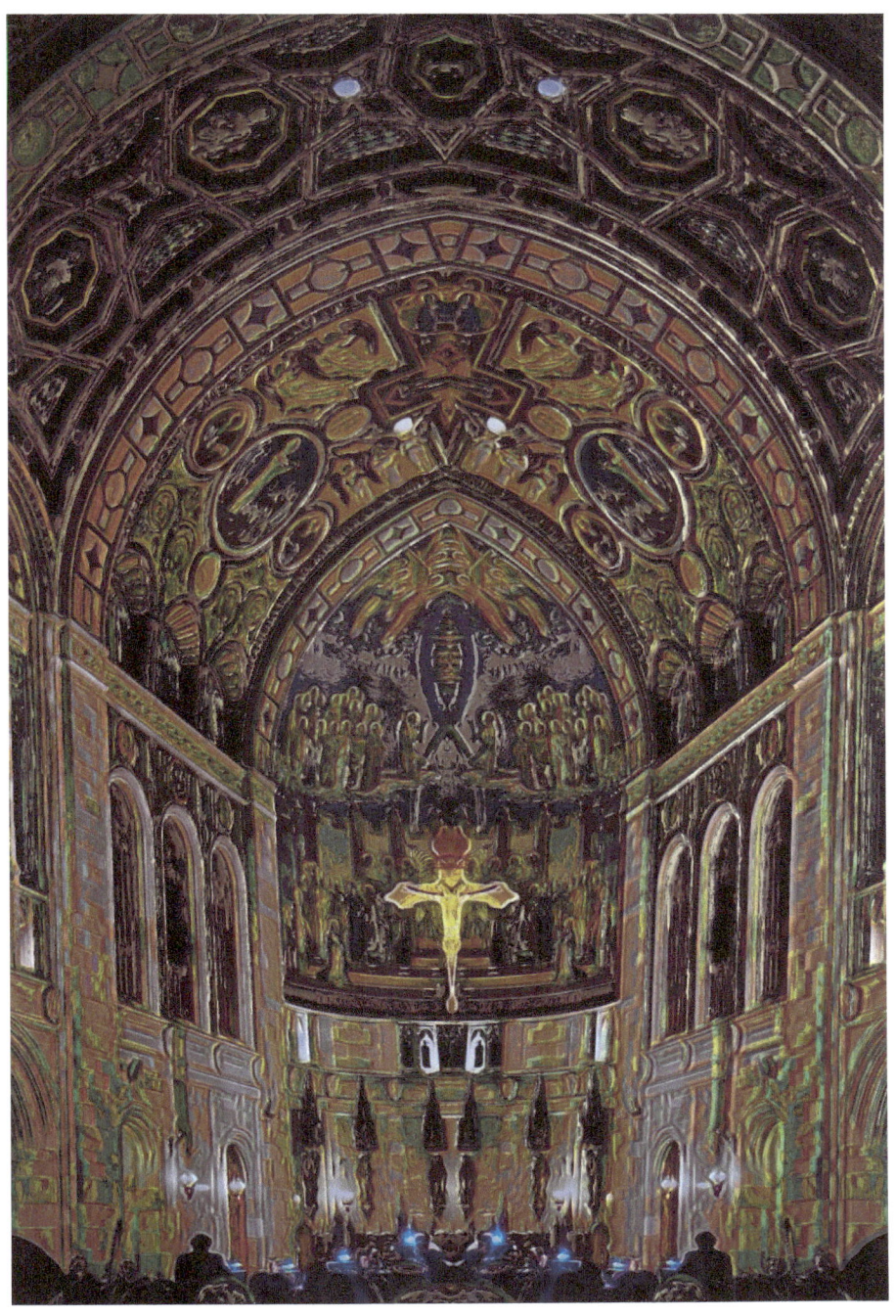

The souls that haunt the mystic ancestry of dreams.

Outis: A Nursing Elegy

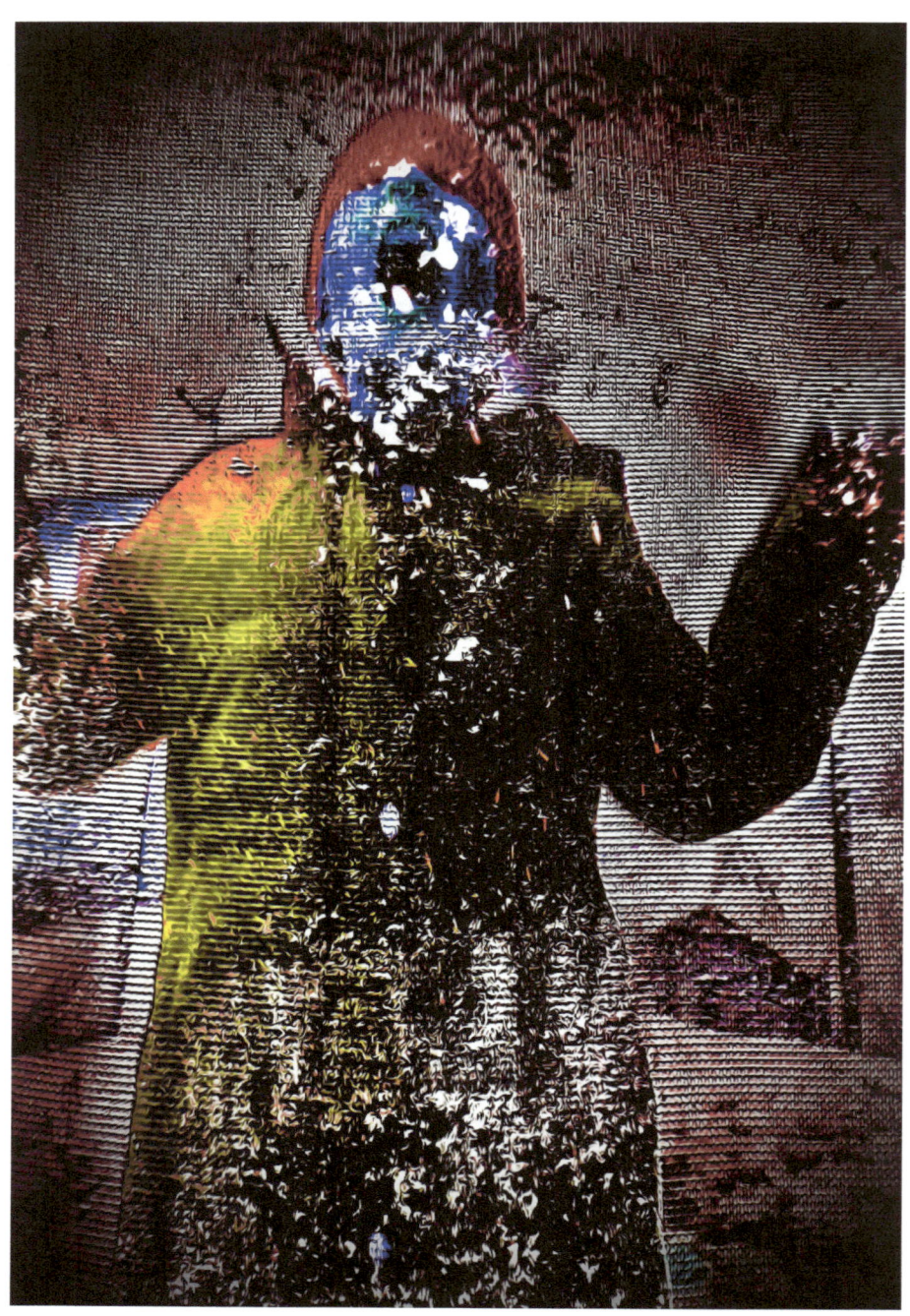

A shifting shade in mood colors all perception;

Outis: A Nursing Elegy

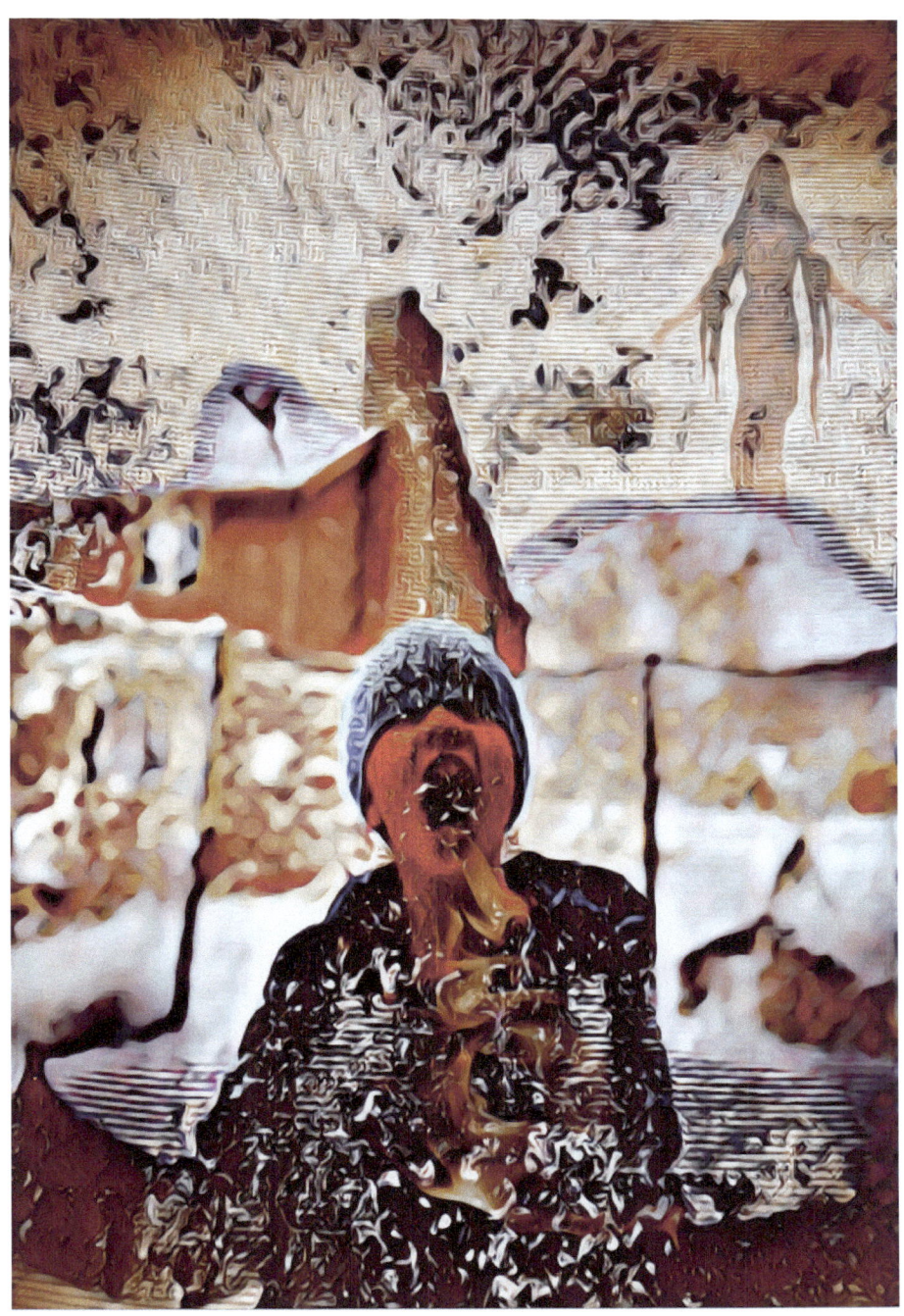

Let them haunt you in the passion of expression.

Outis: A Nursing Elegy

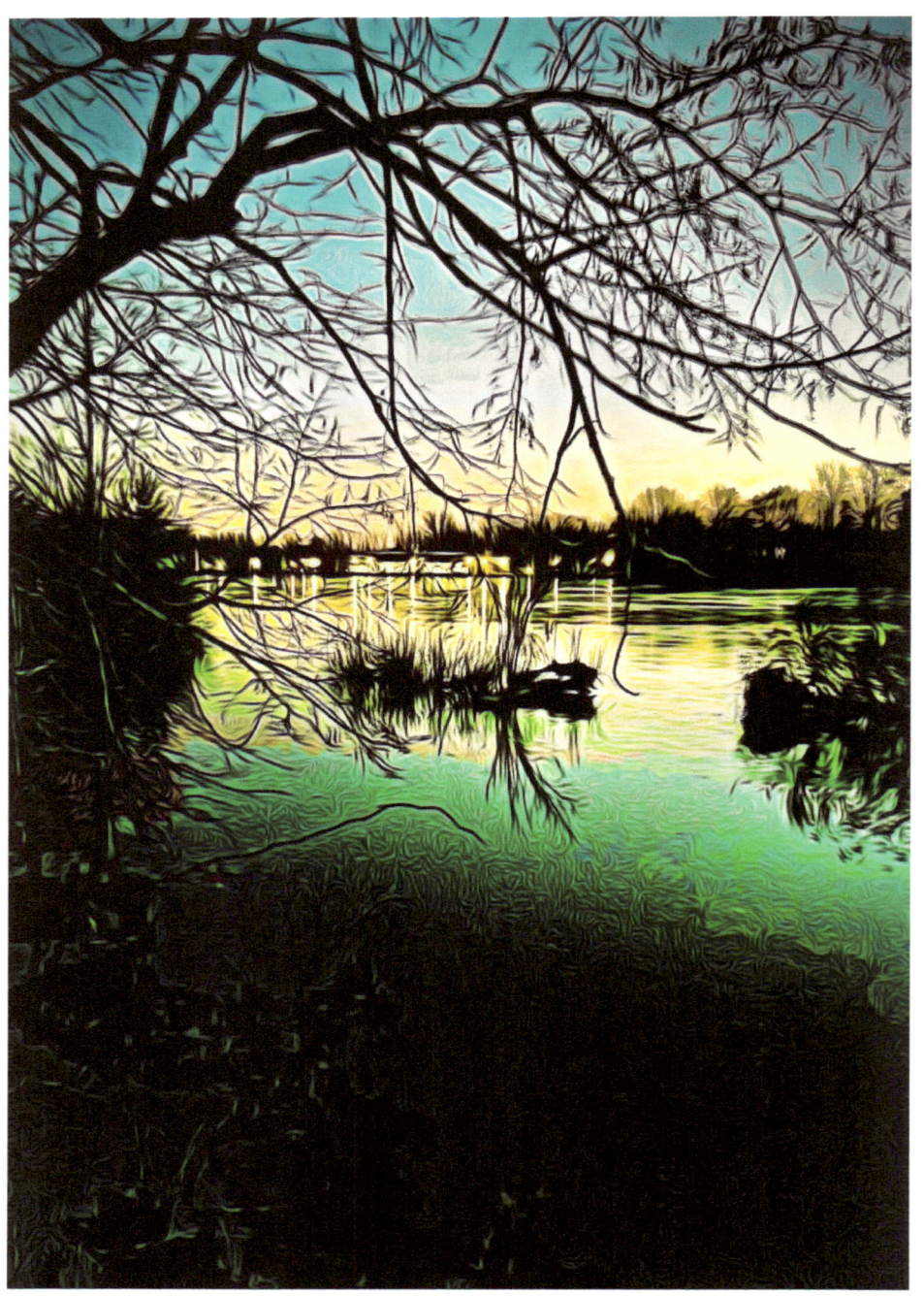

The stormy mist and frost kiss on fresh-fallen leaves.

Outis: A Nursing Elegy

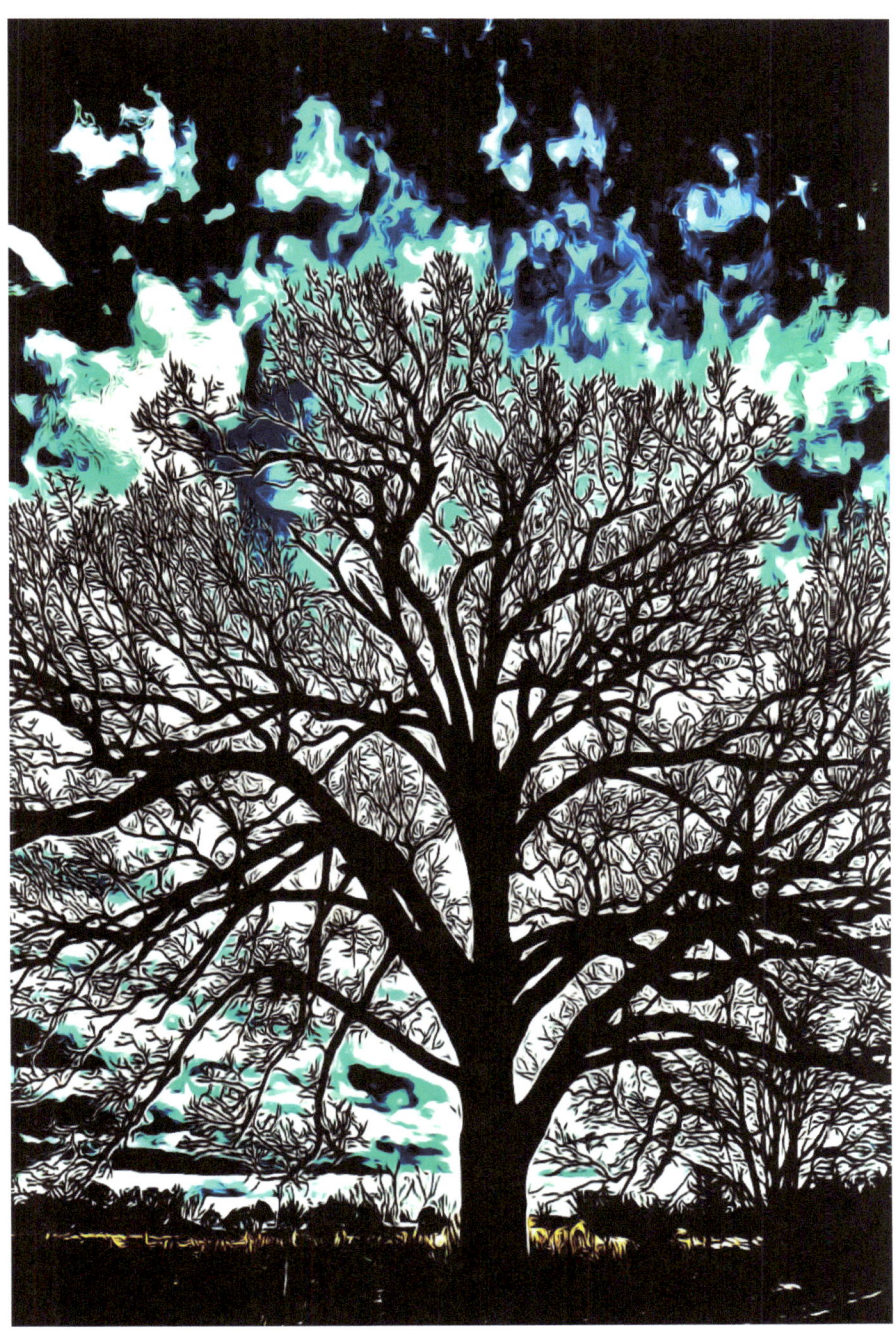

The moaning breeze cracking the shriveled tree fingers.

Outis: A Nursing Elegy

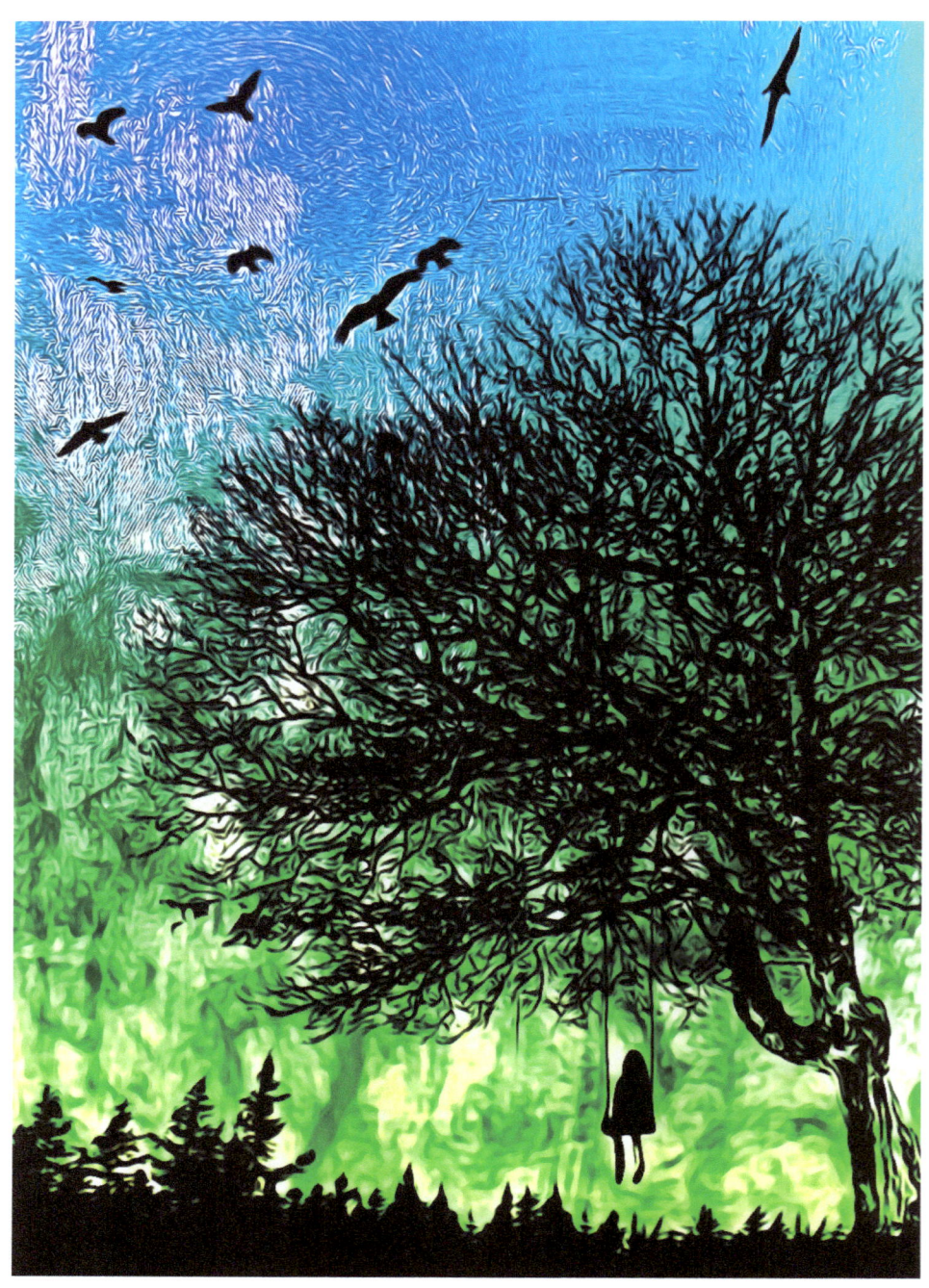

Nature manifests metaphors for those that grieve . . .

Outis: A Nursing Elegy

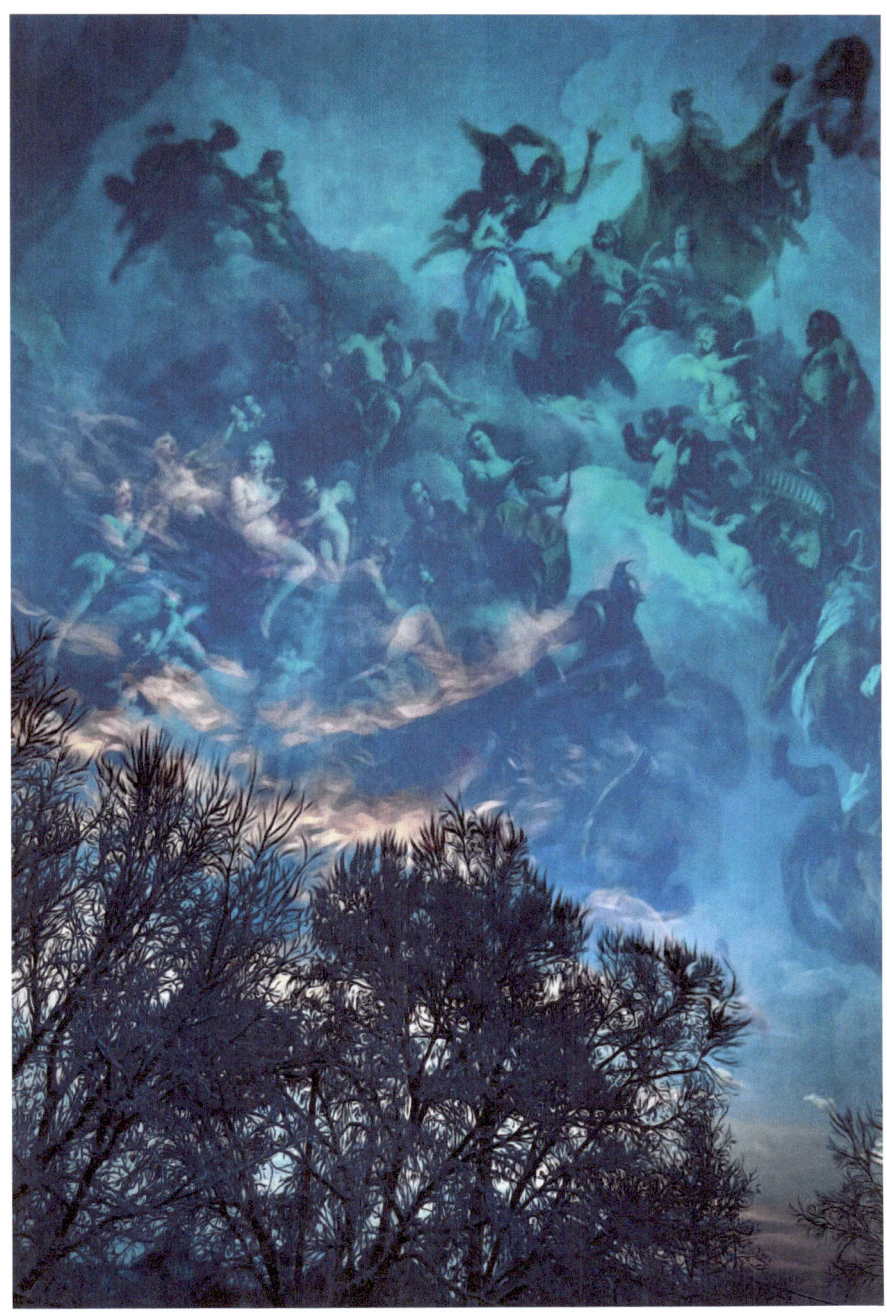

What is there for those who know the passing spirits

Outis: A Nursing Elegy

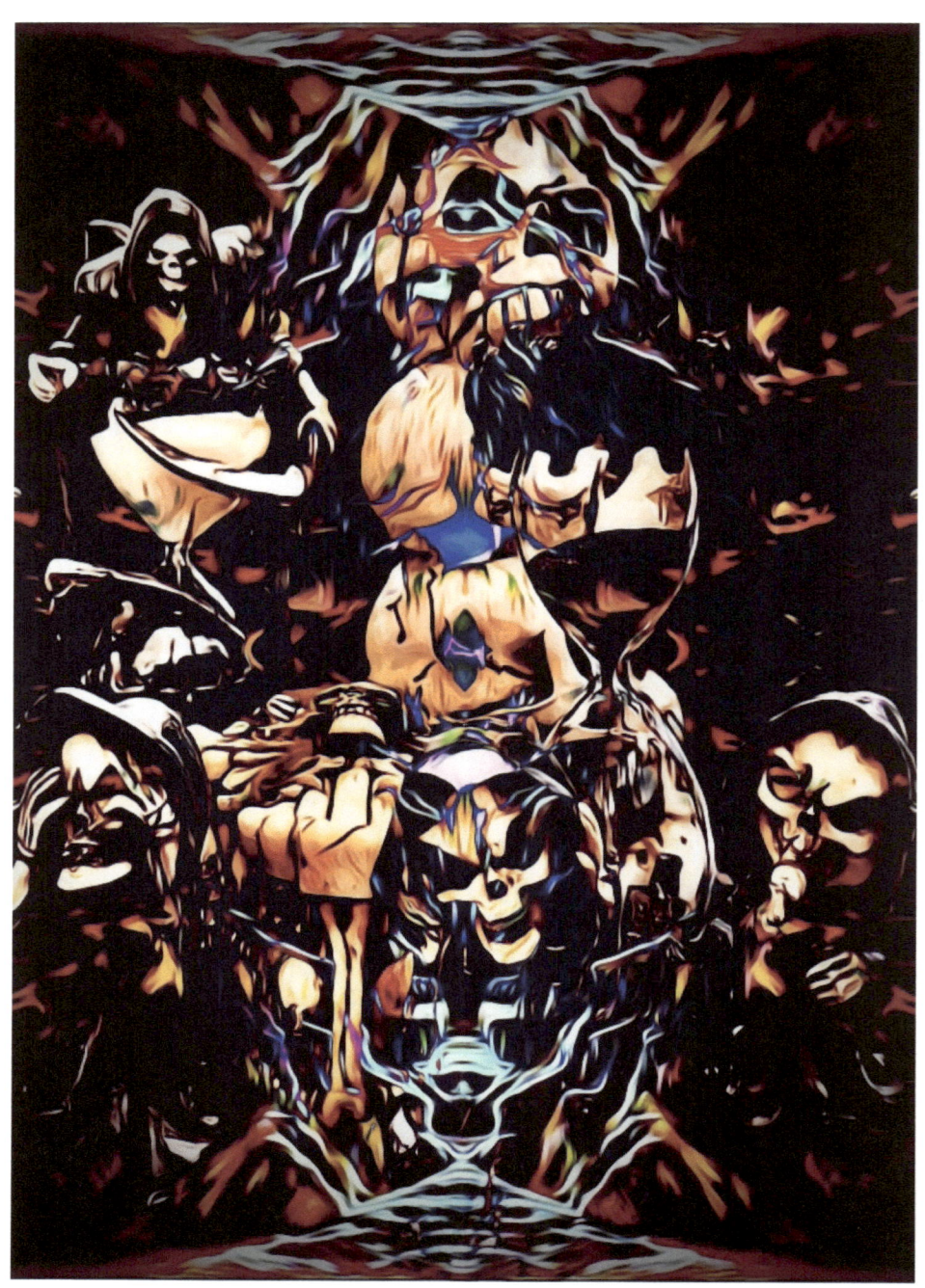

But not how the departed lived?

Outis: A Nursing Elegy

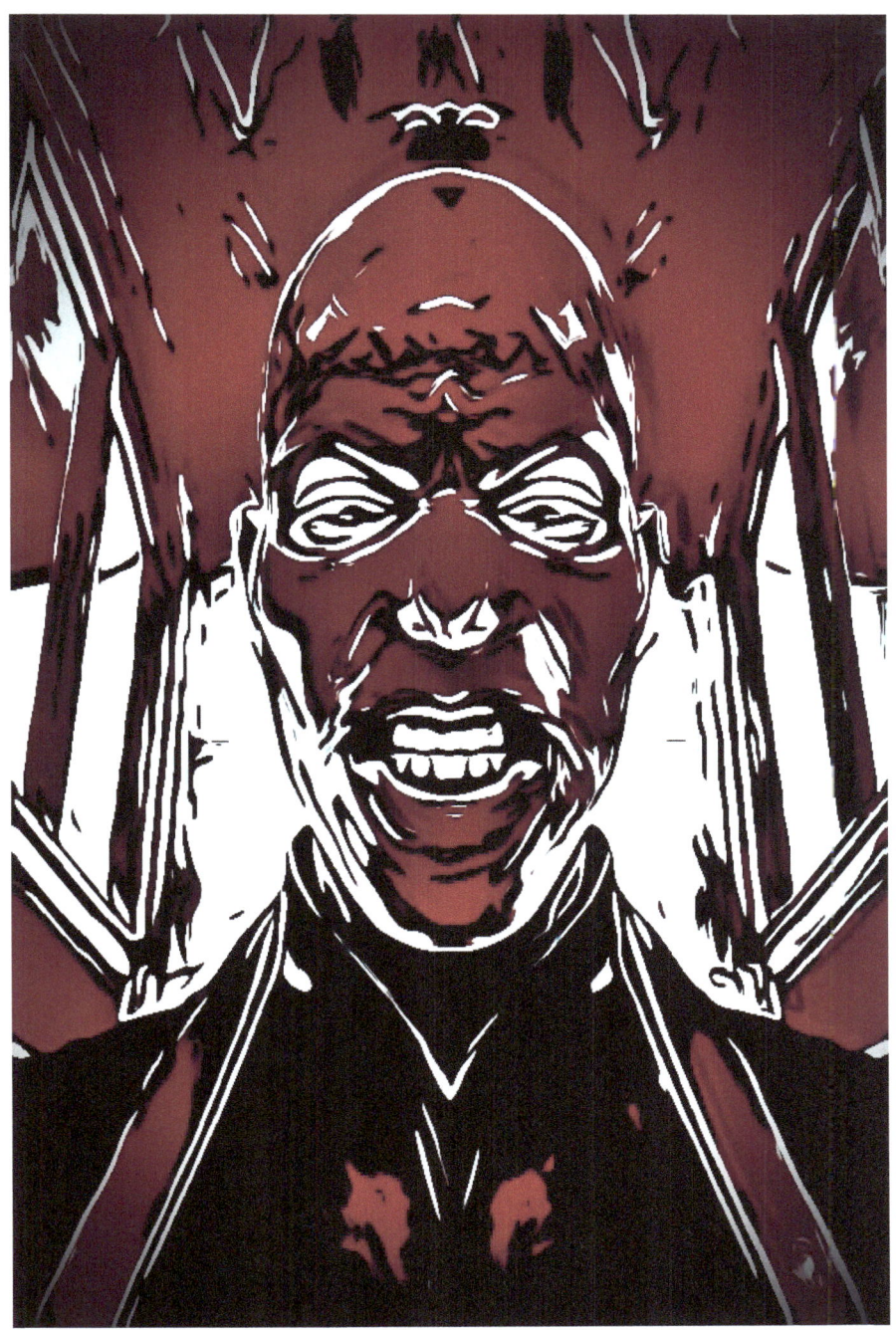

How death lingers

Outis: A Nursing Elegy

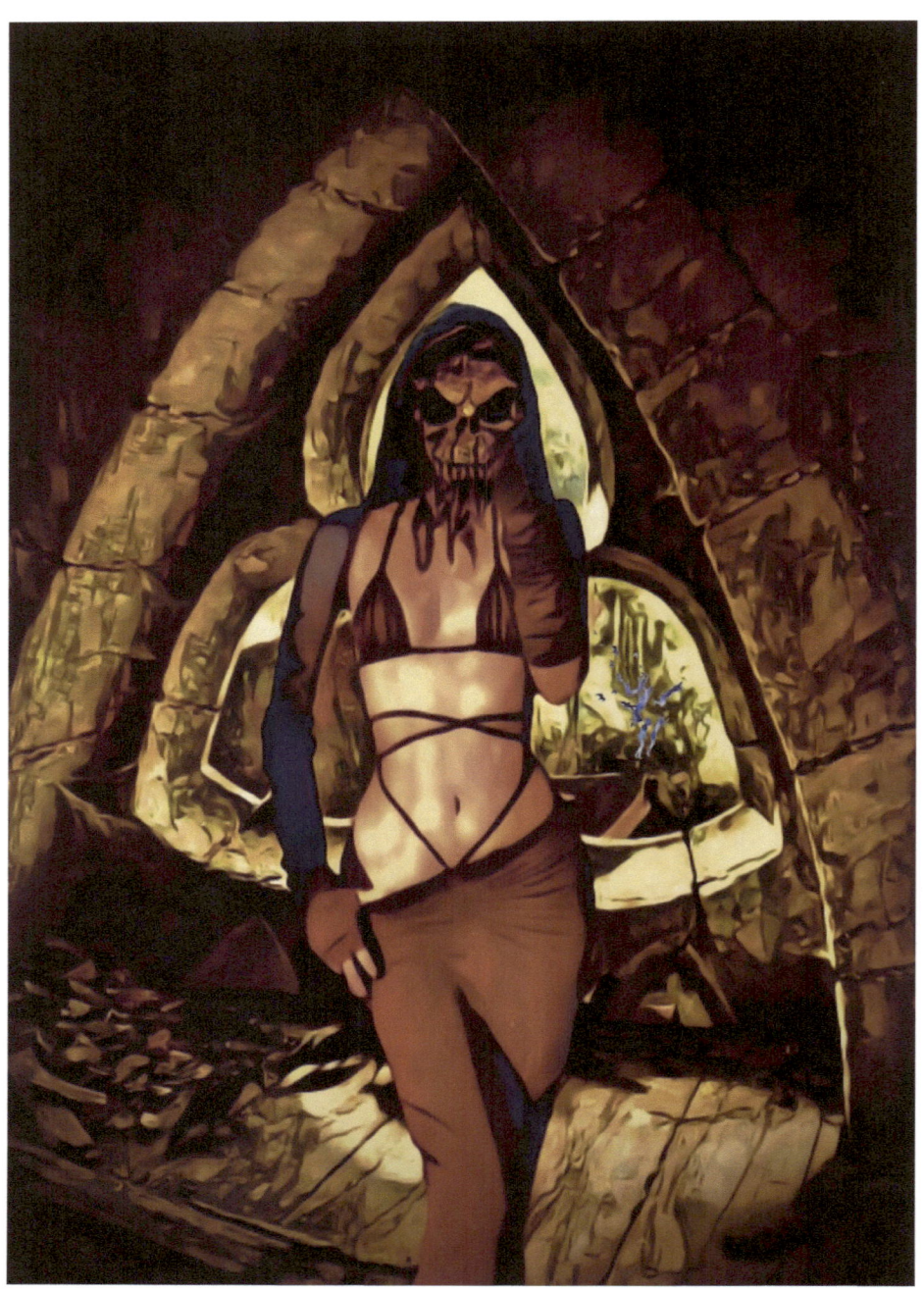

In beds, in rooms that other souls must inherit.

Outis: A Nursing Elegy

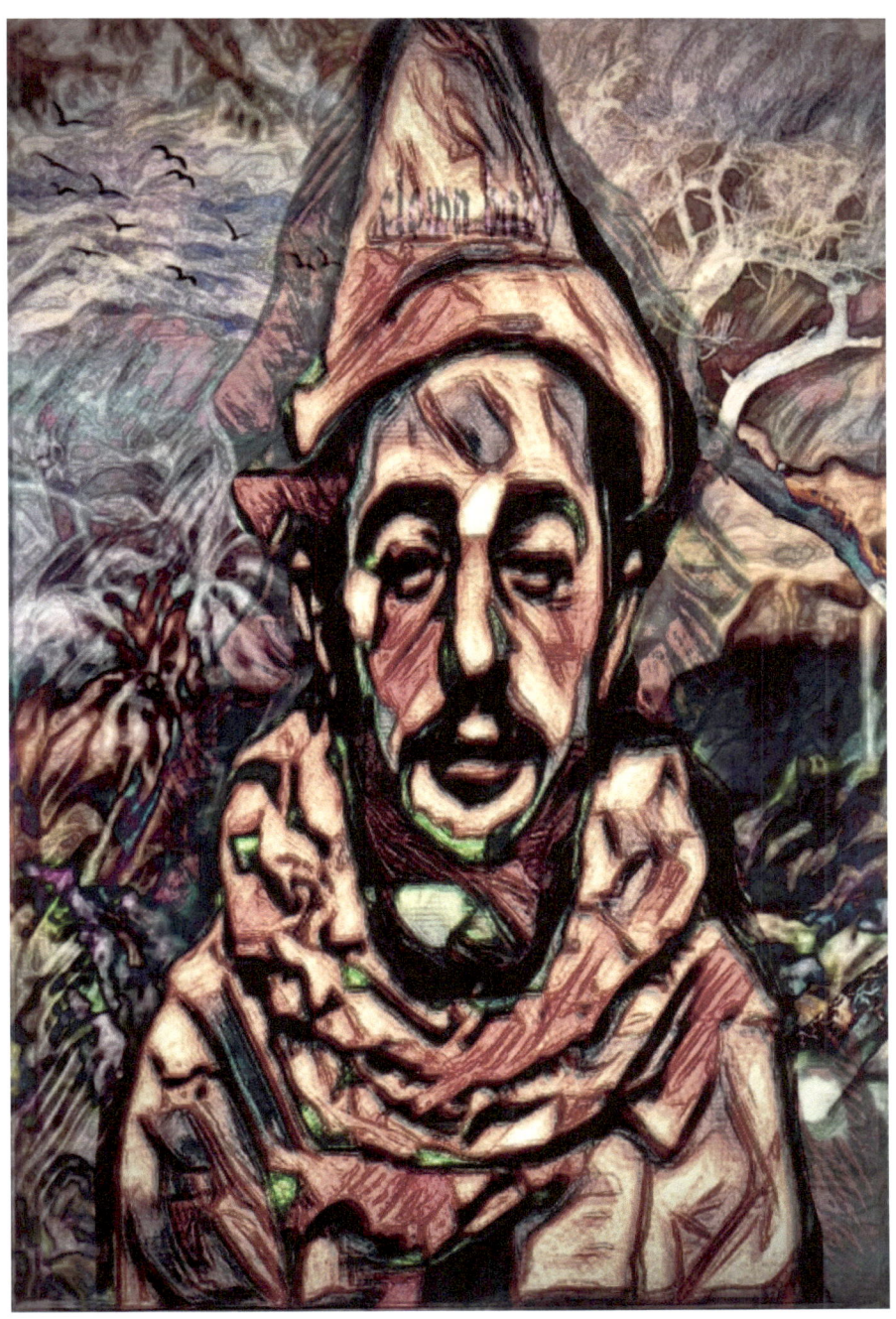

Names fade from consciousness. -

Outis: A Nursing Elegy

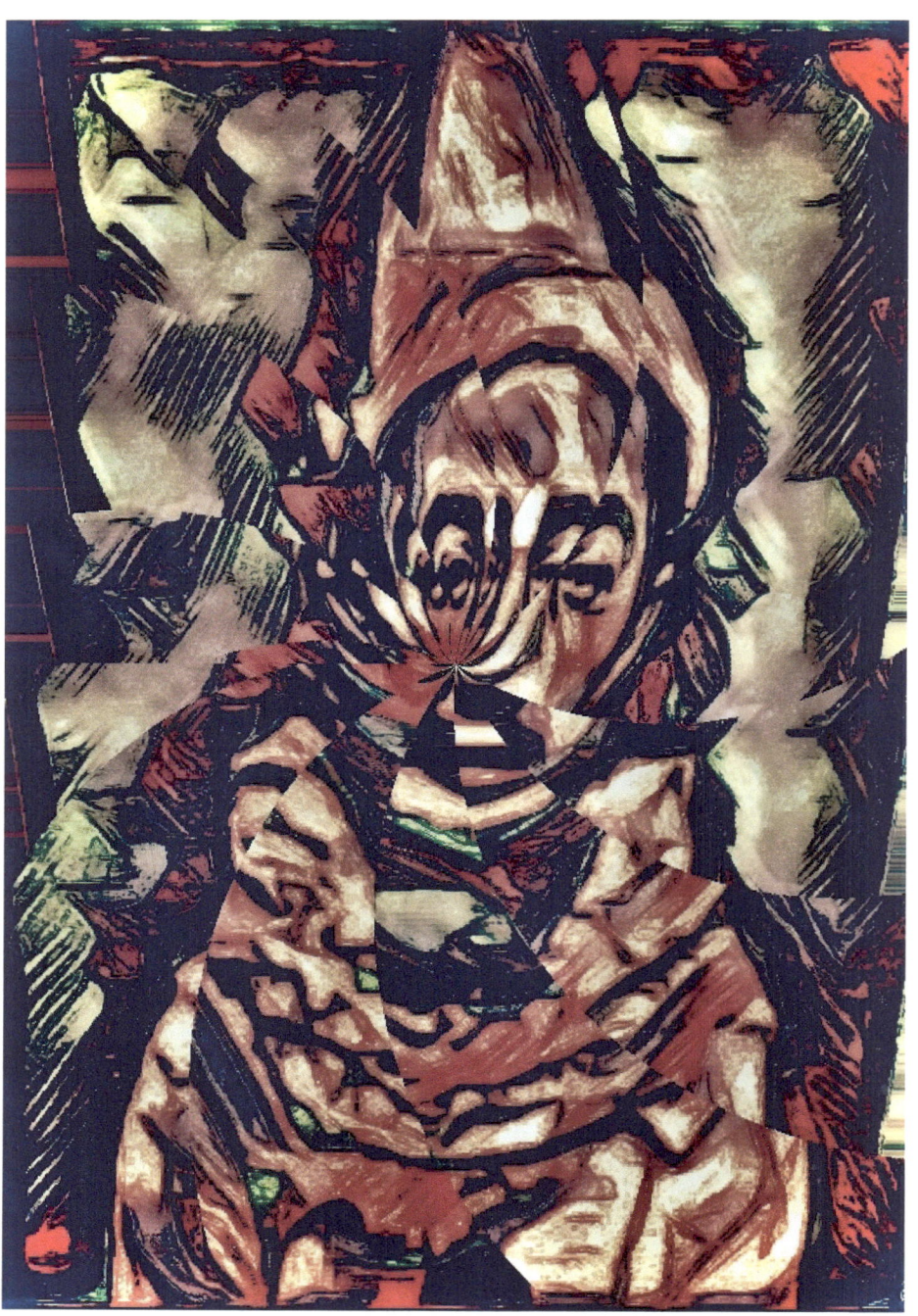

The fates become destined. -

Outis: A Nursing Elegy

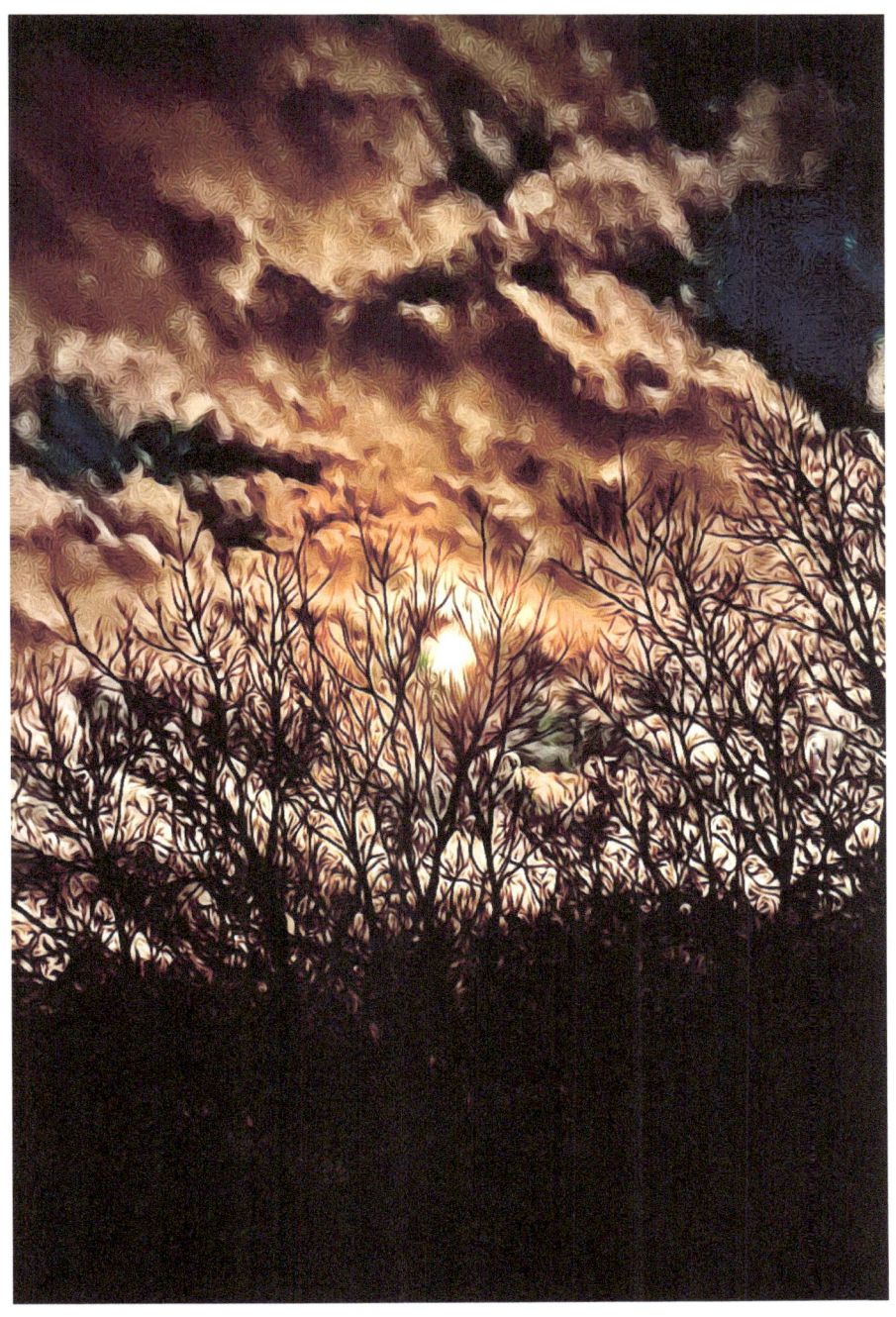

While the life-uprising against death soldiers on.

Outis: A Nursing Elegy

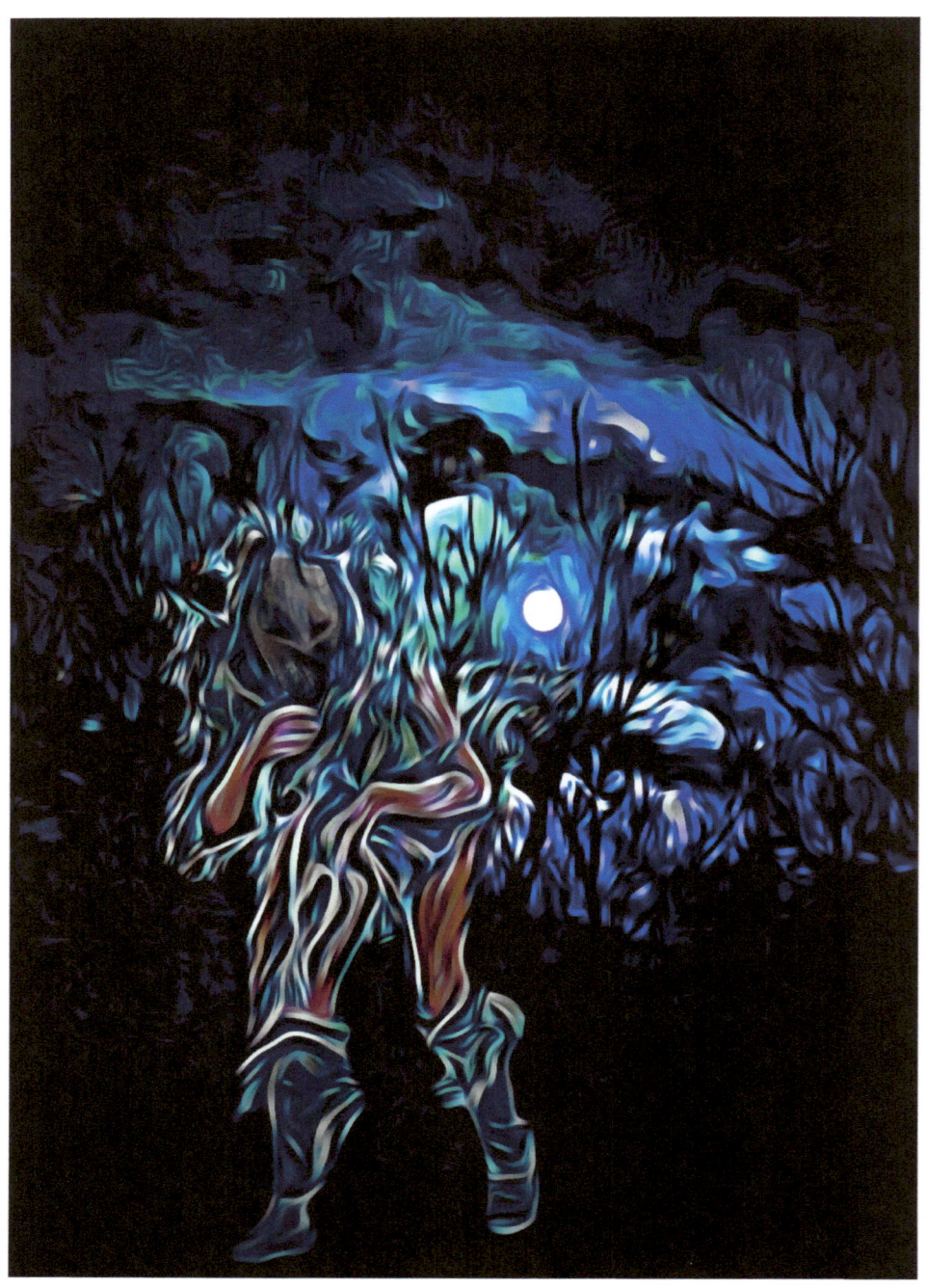

Then a haunting flashes those of final blessings-

Outis: A Nursing Elegy

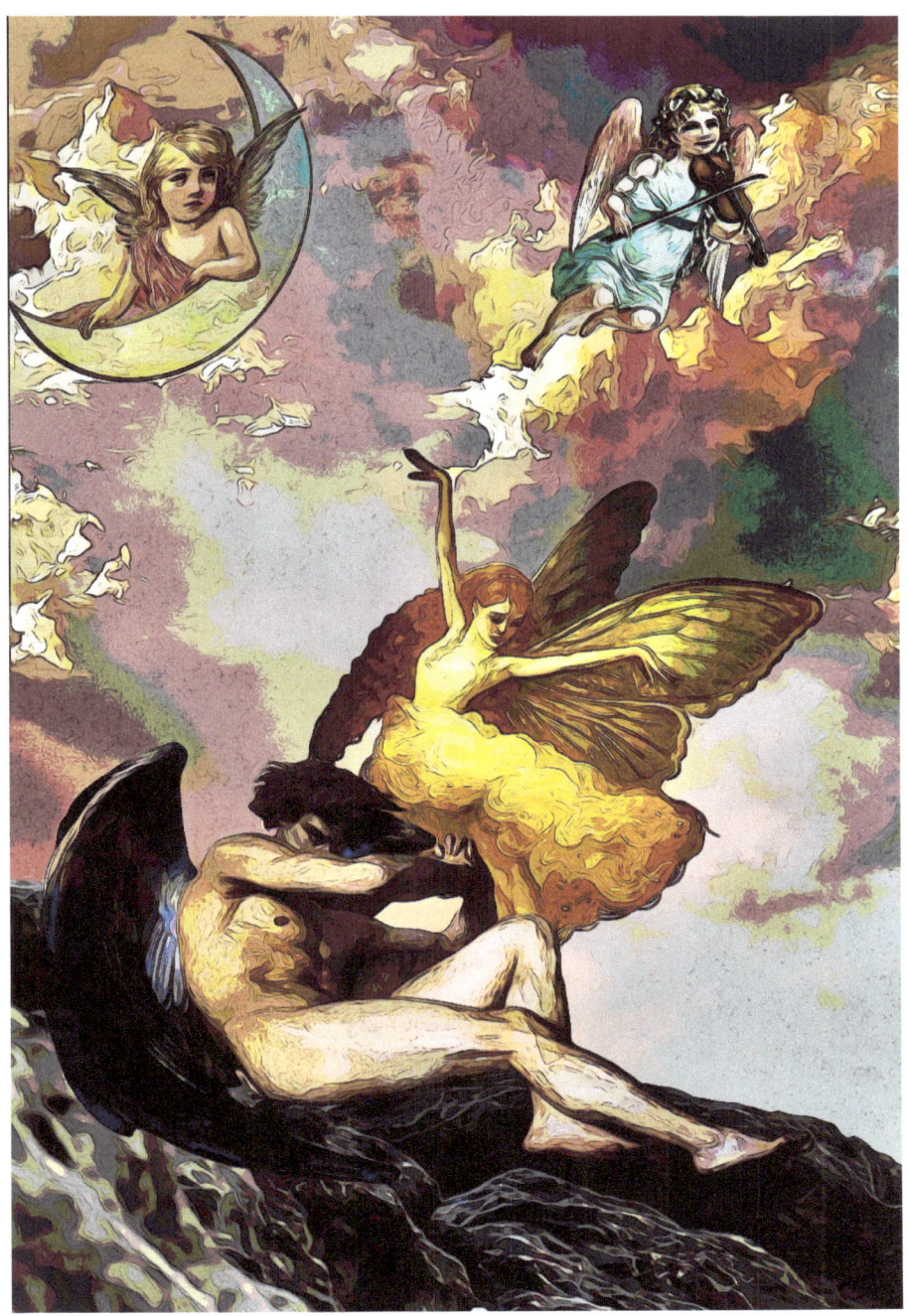

The defeat of knowing,

Outis: A Nursing Elegy

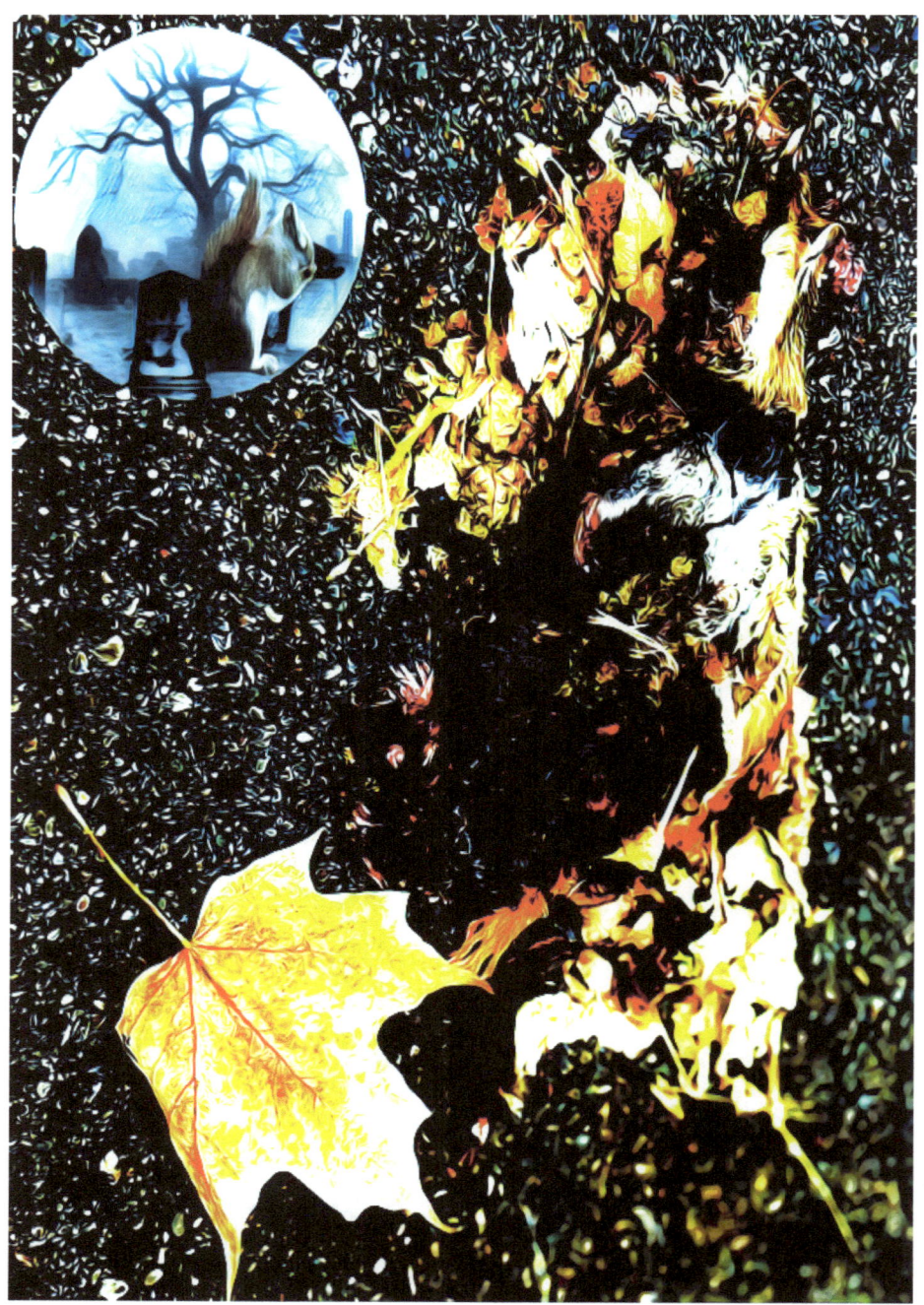

The gasp of agony-

Outis: A Nursing Elegy

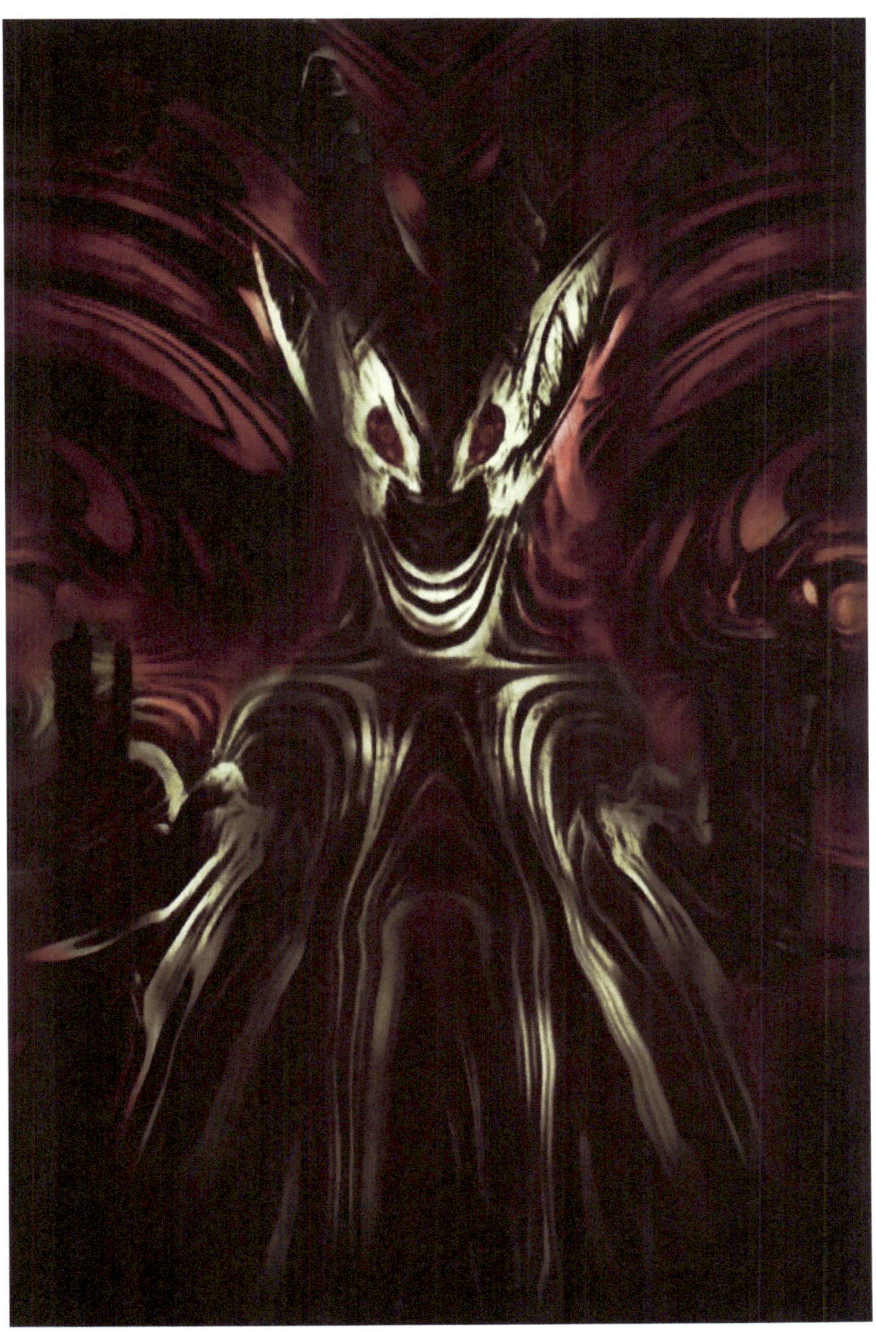

(Breaths of truths no one can divulge into a song.) -

Outis: A Nursing Elegy

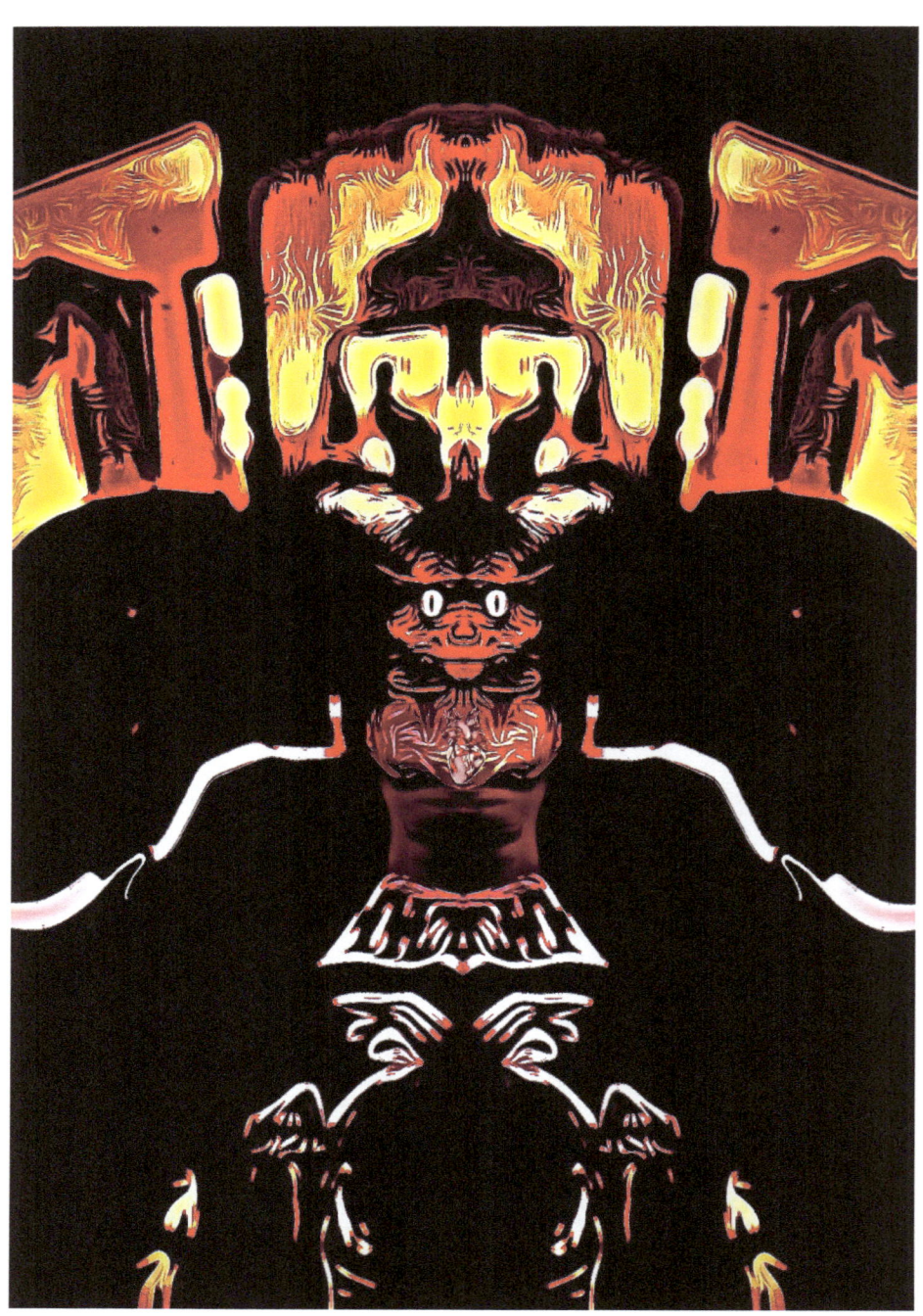

To shed light on tragedies of reality:

Outis: A Nursing Elegy

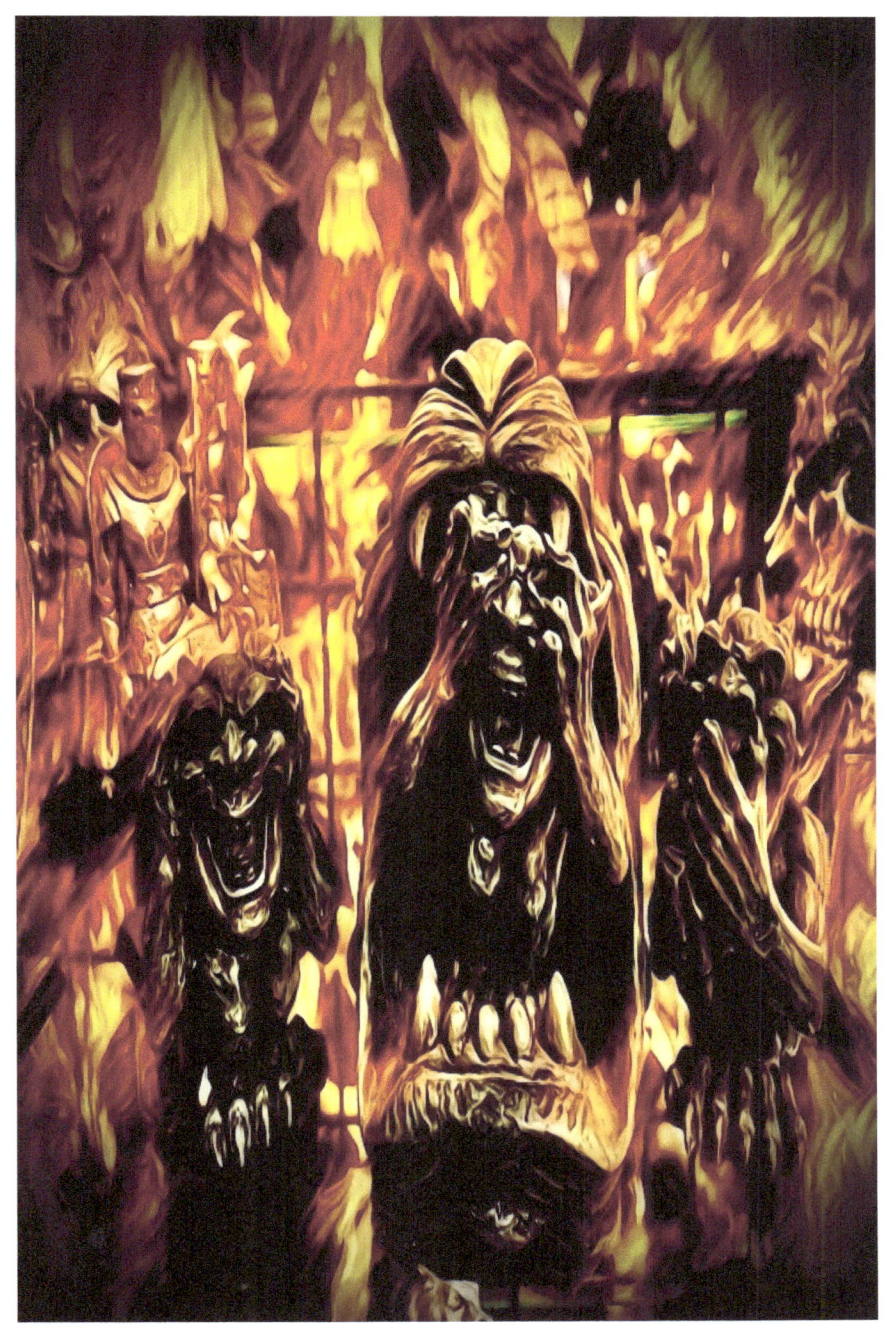

Those that witness can only own experience.

Outis: A Nursing Elegy

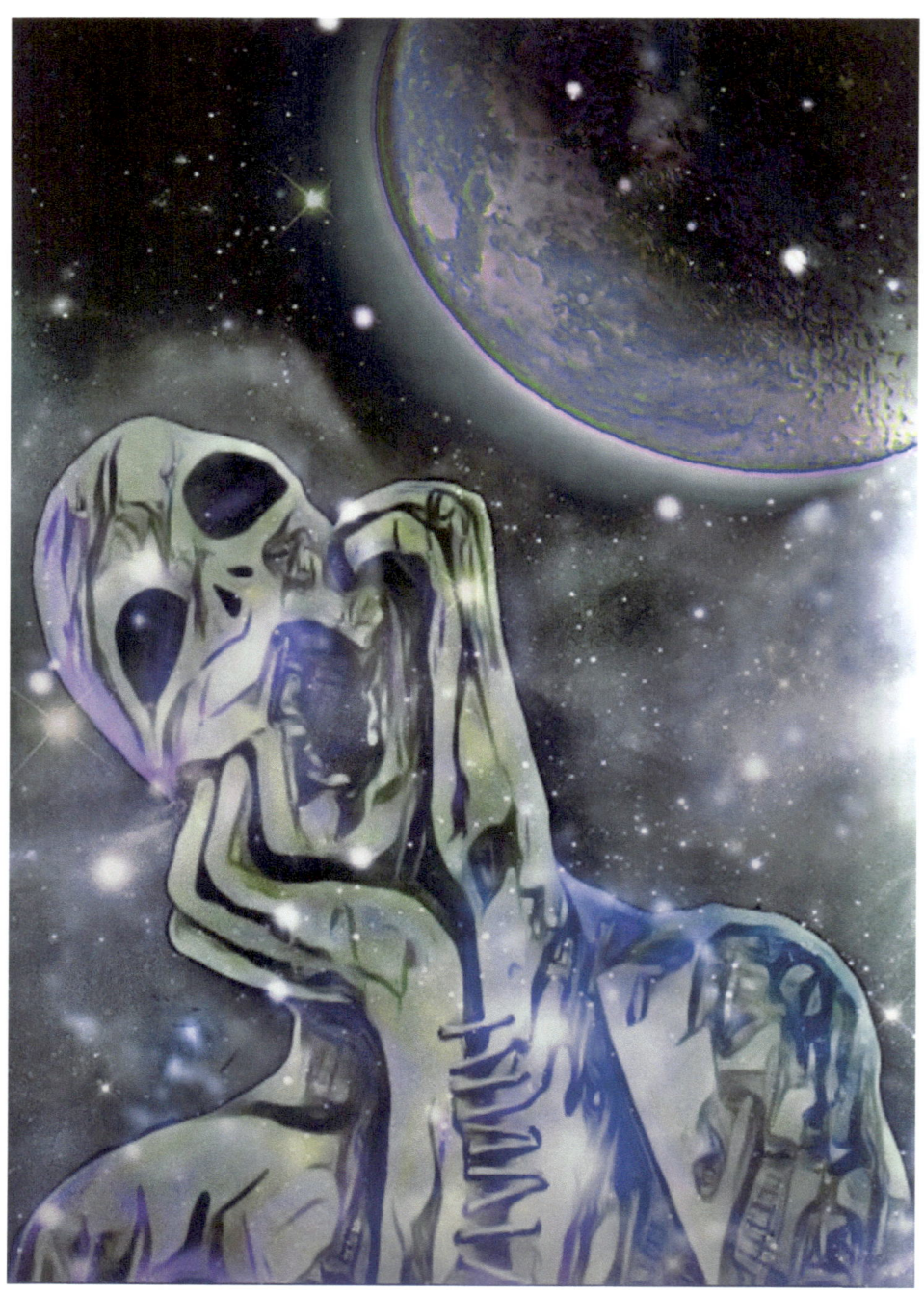

One must decide if that's a curse or providence.

Outis: A Nursing Elegy

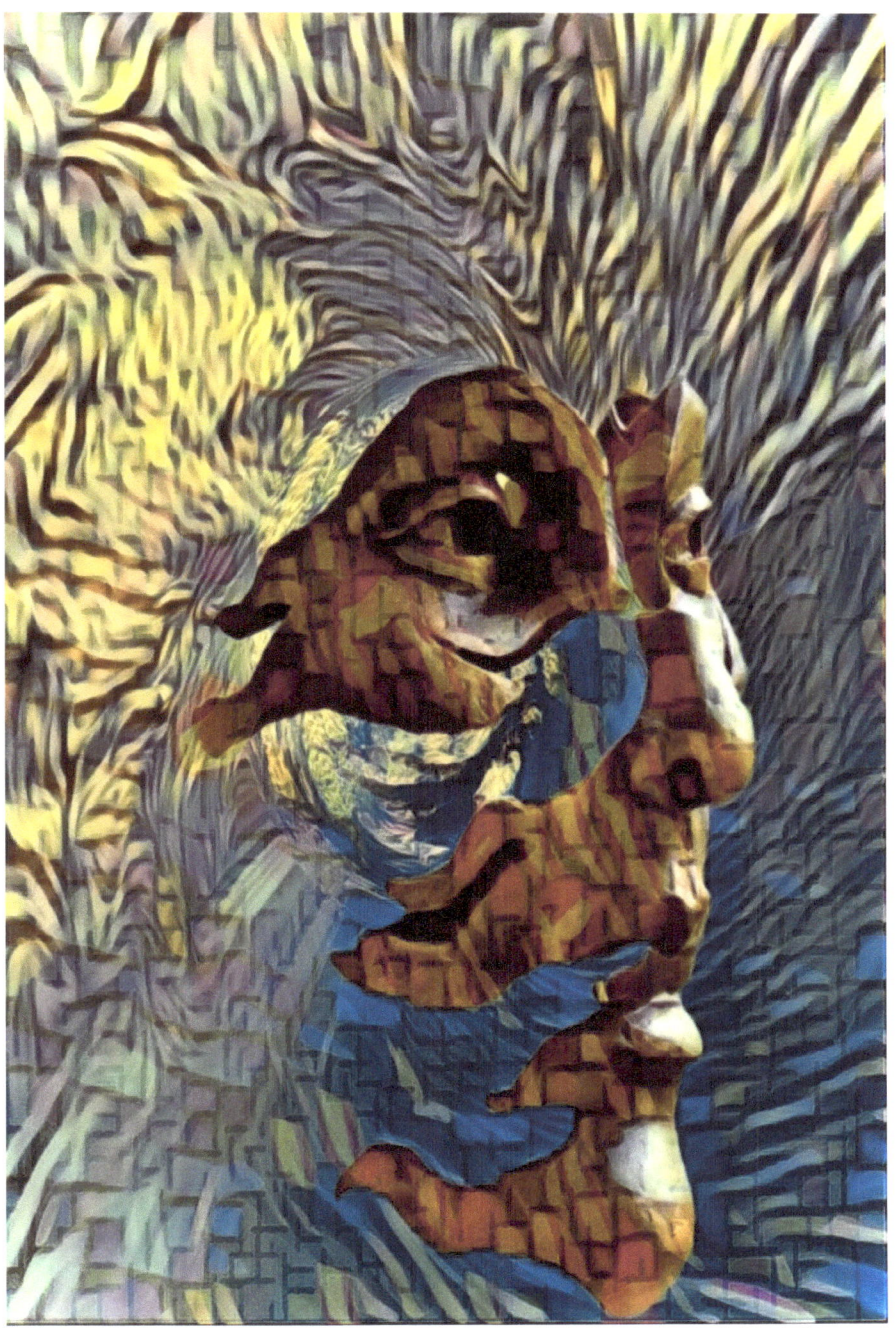

The winds of grief whistle through the reeds of requiem.

Outis: A Nursing Elegy

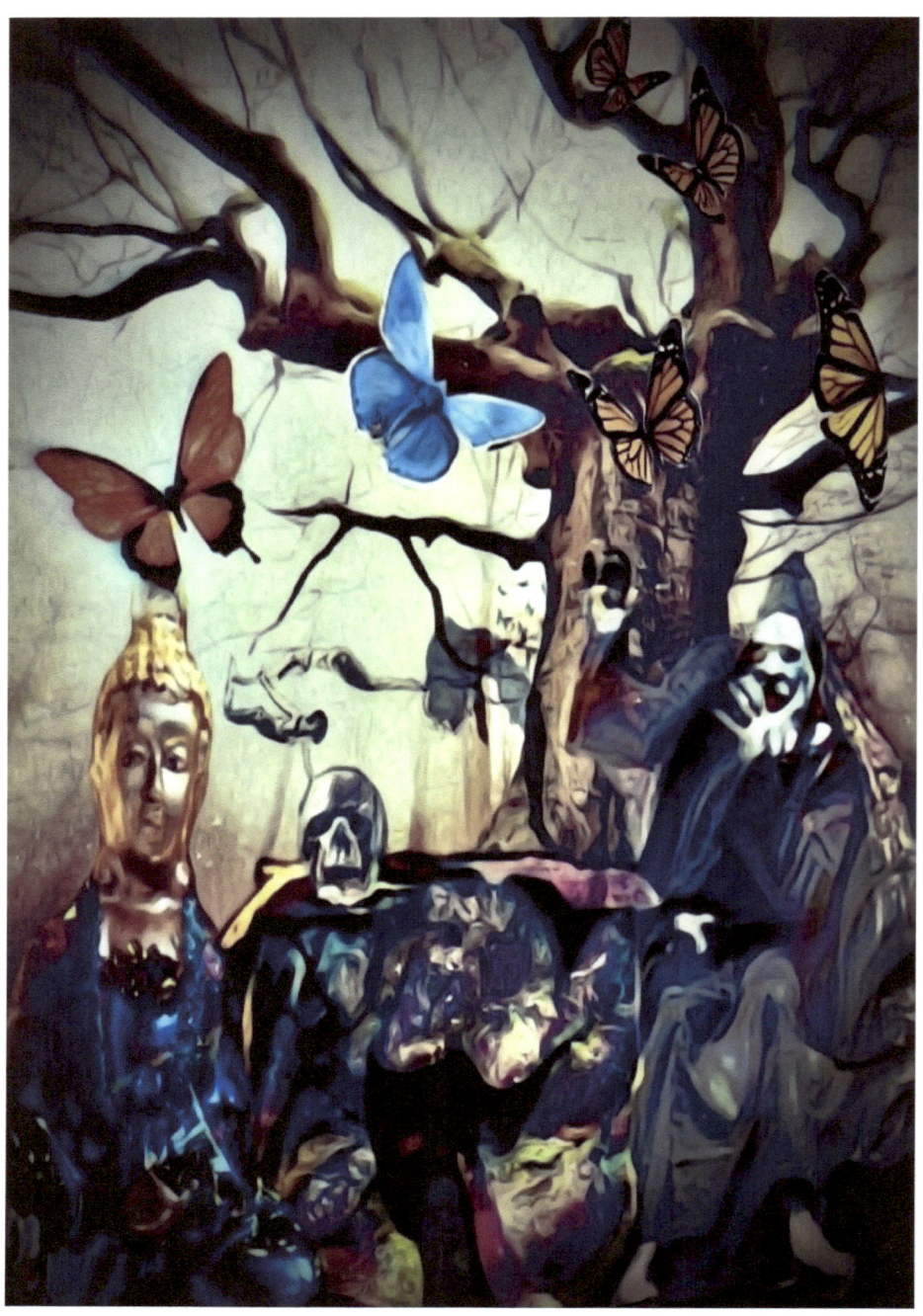

Summer leaves become autumn gold and then take leave.

Outis: A Nursing Elegy

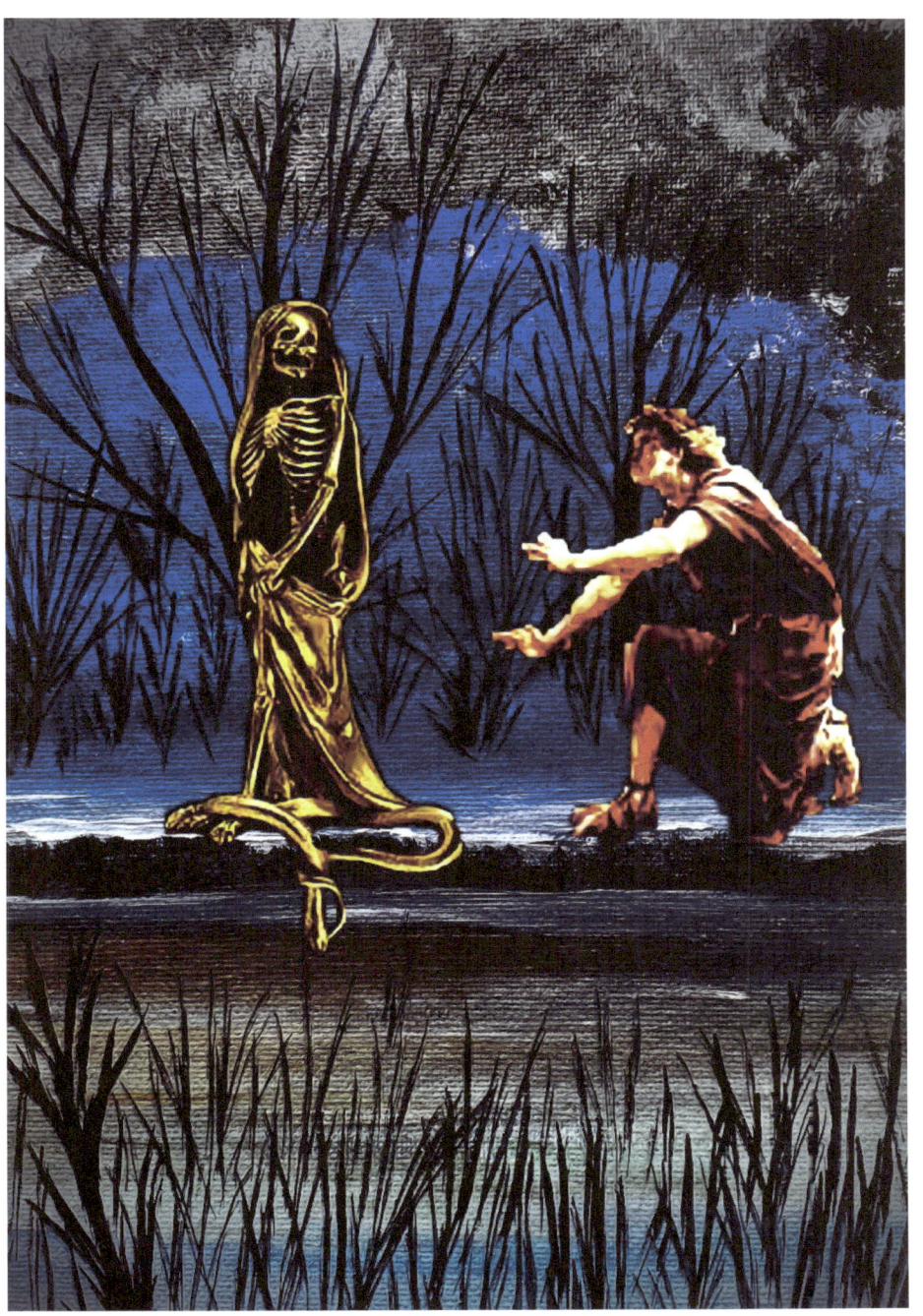

The winter-today hardens phantoms of ransom. . .

Outis: A Nursing Elegy

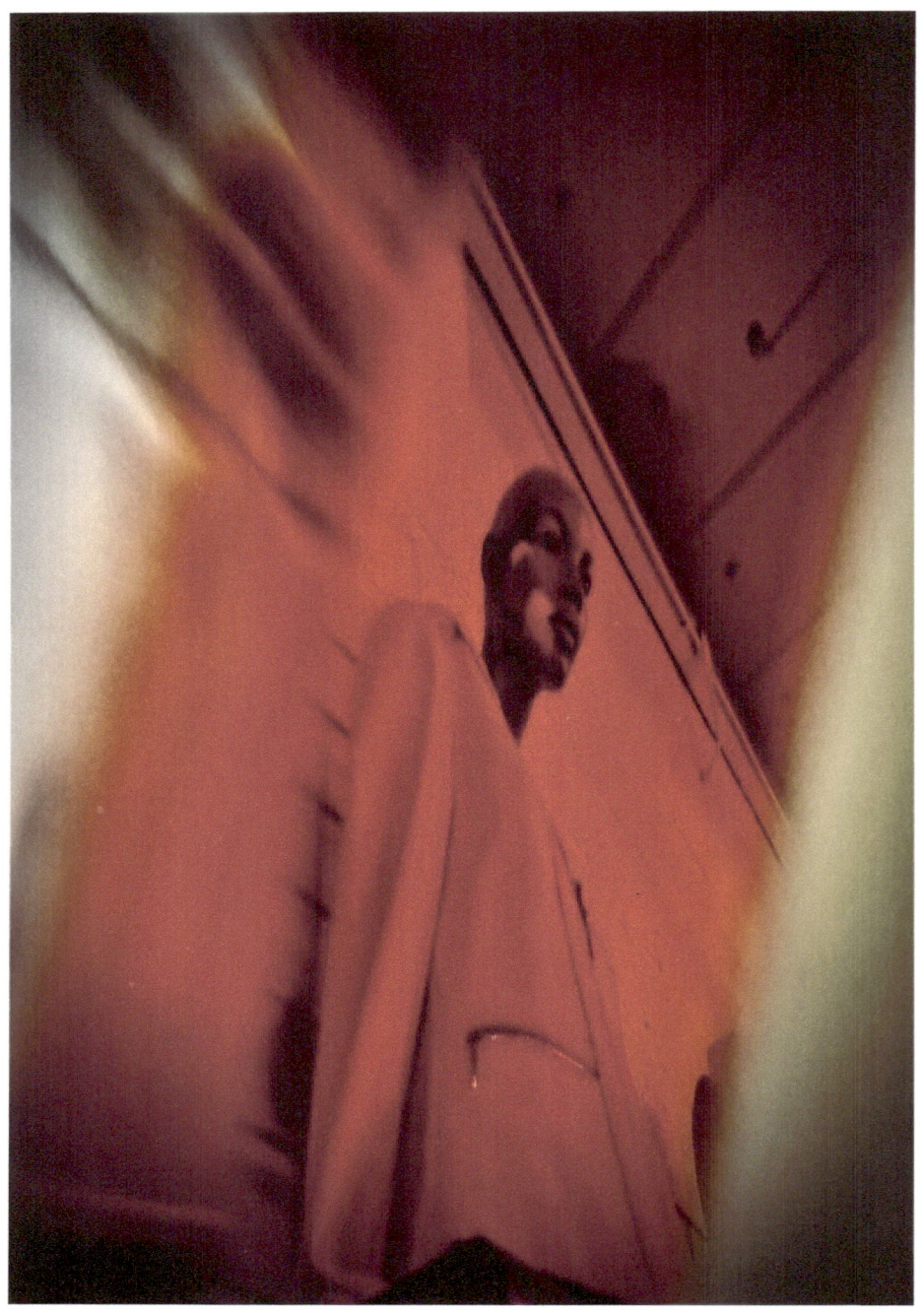

The charlatans try to ensure you in their wares

Outis: A Nursing Elegy

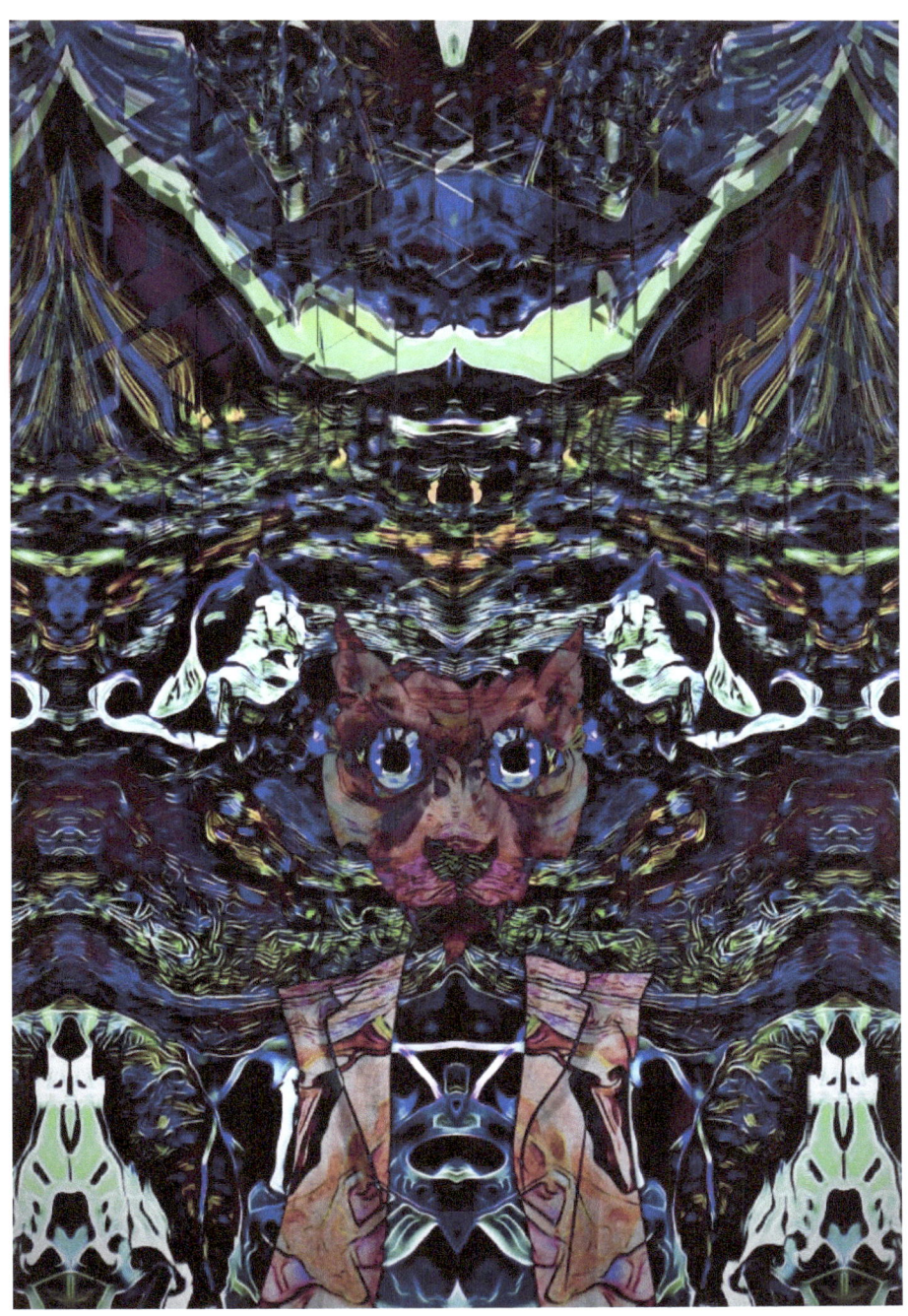

To become a lotus eater that never grieves

Outis: A Nursing Elegy

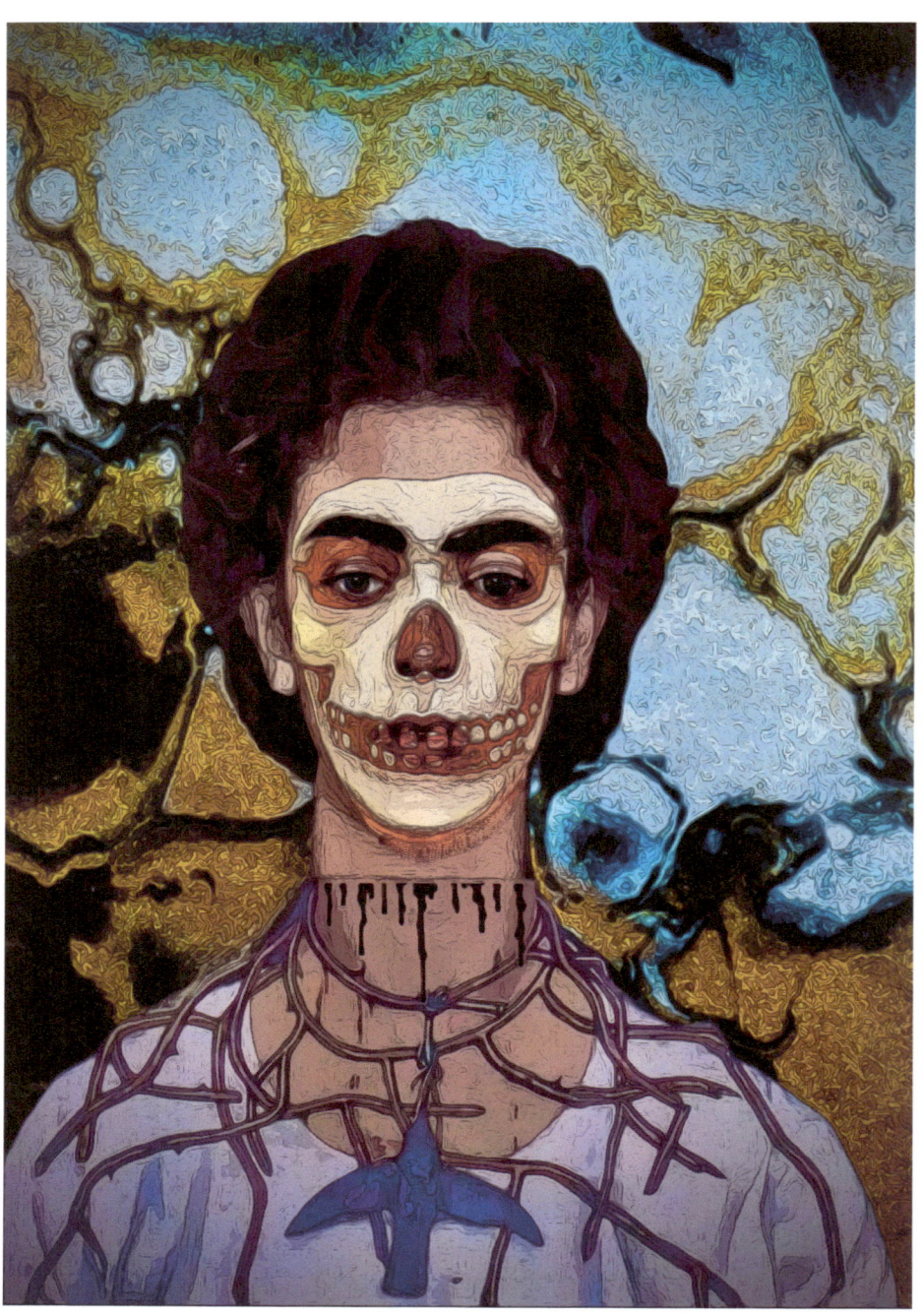

The war fallen and those causes left unaware.

Outis: A Nursing Elegy

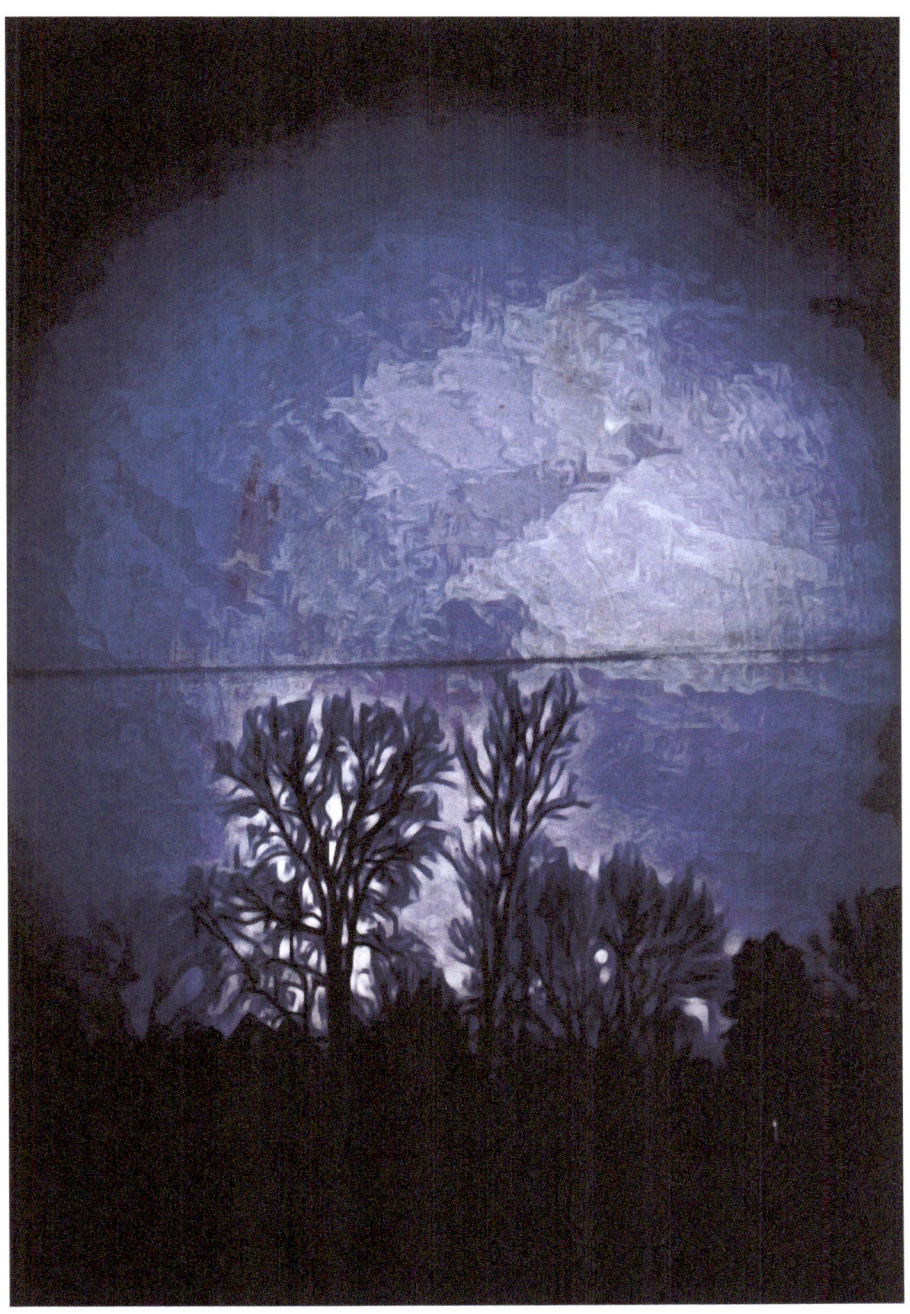

And, although we are never found, we are not lost...

Outis: A Nursing Elegy

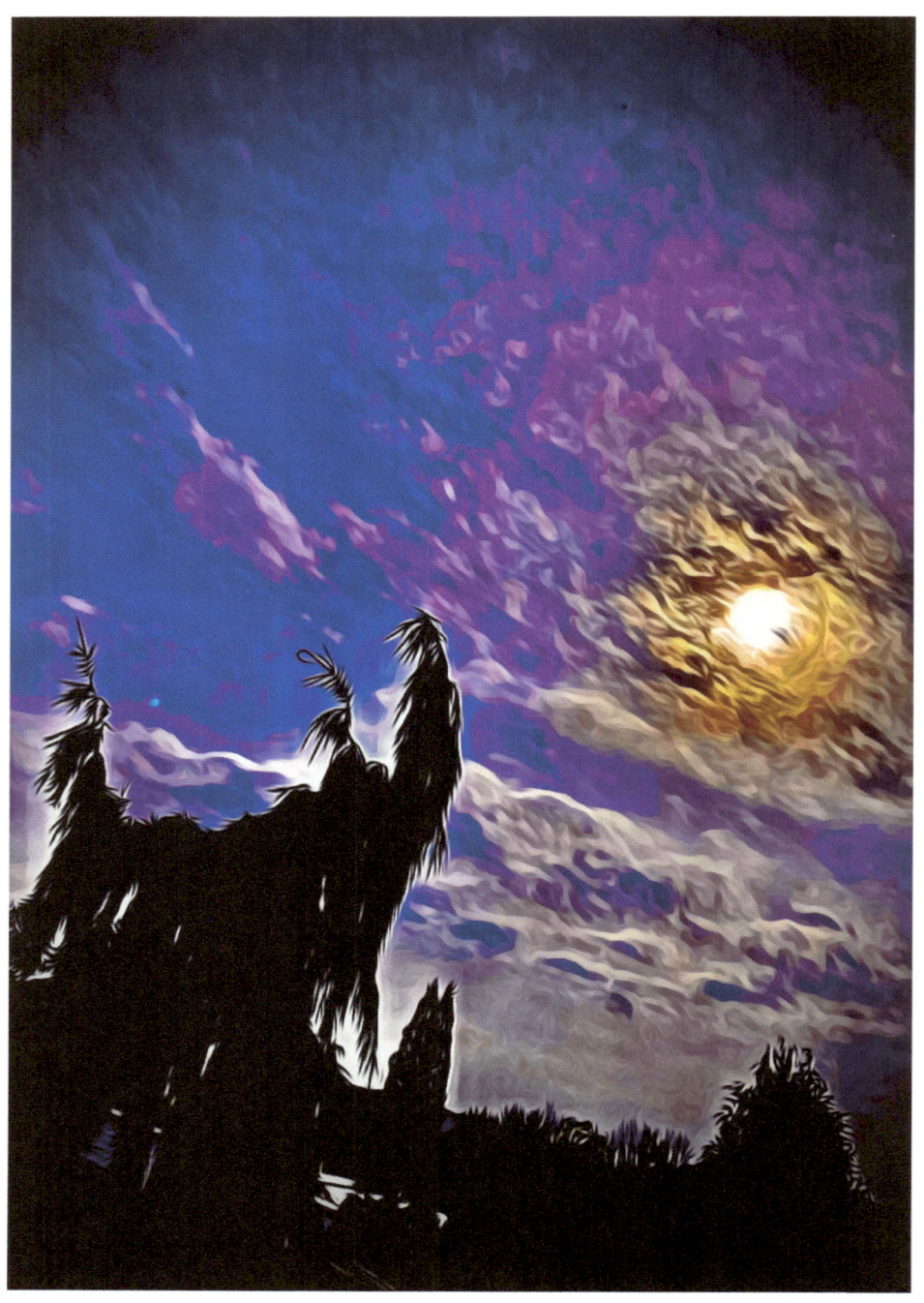

A loneliness among the beauty of nature,

Outis: A Nursing Elegy

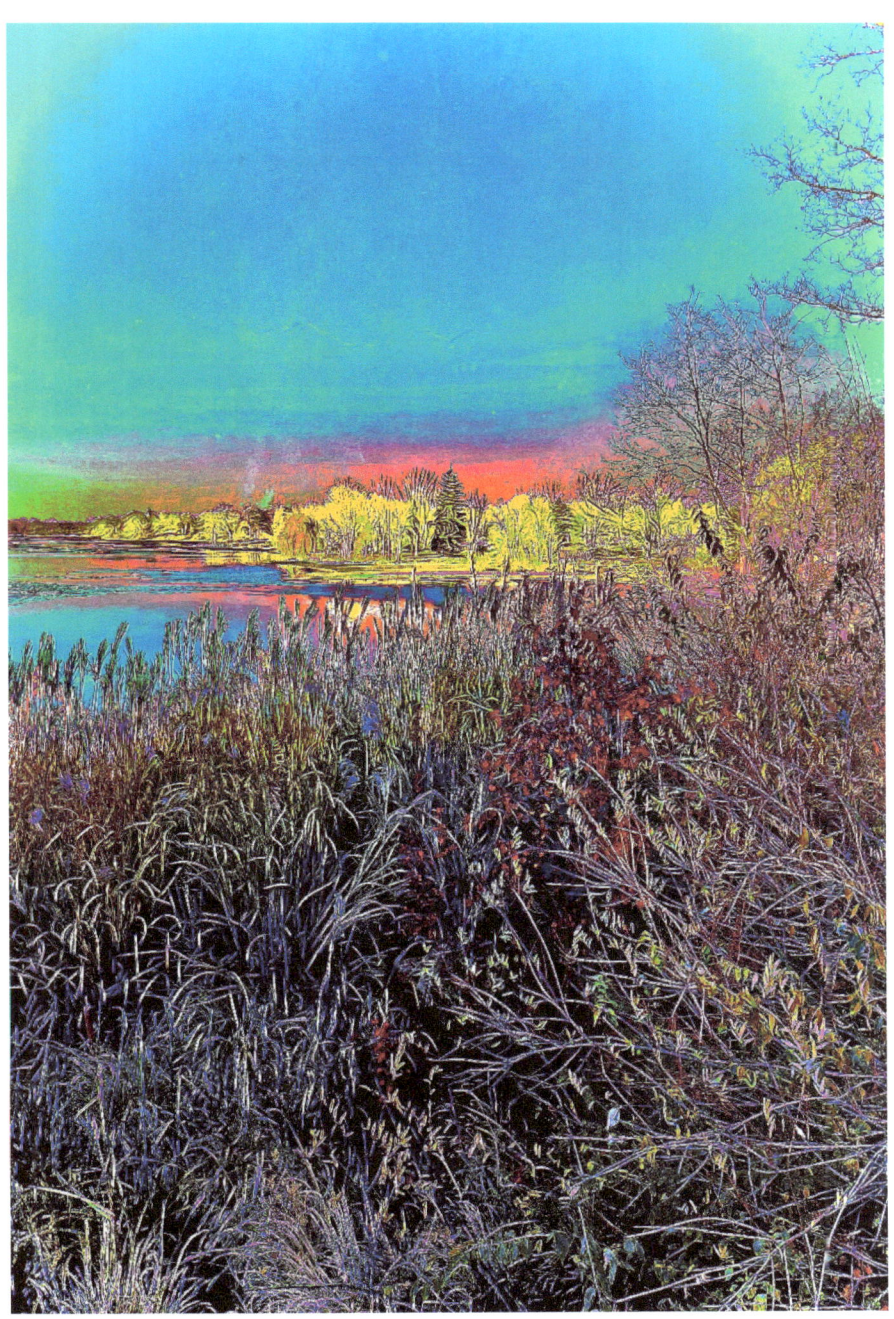

The odd shift in seasonal patterns- that's the cost.

Outis: A Nursing Elegy

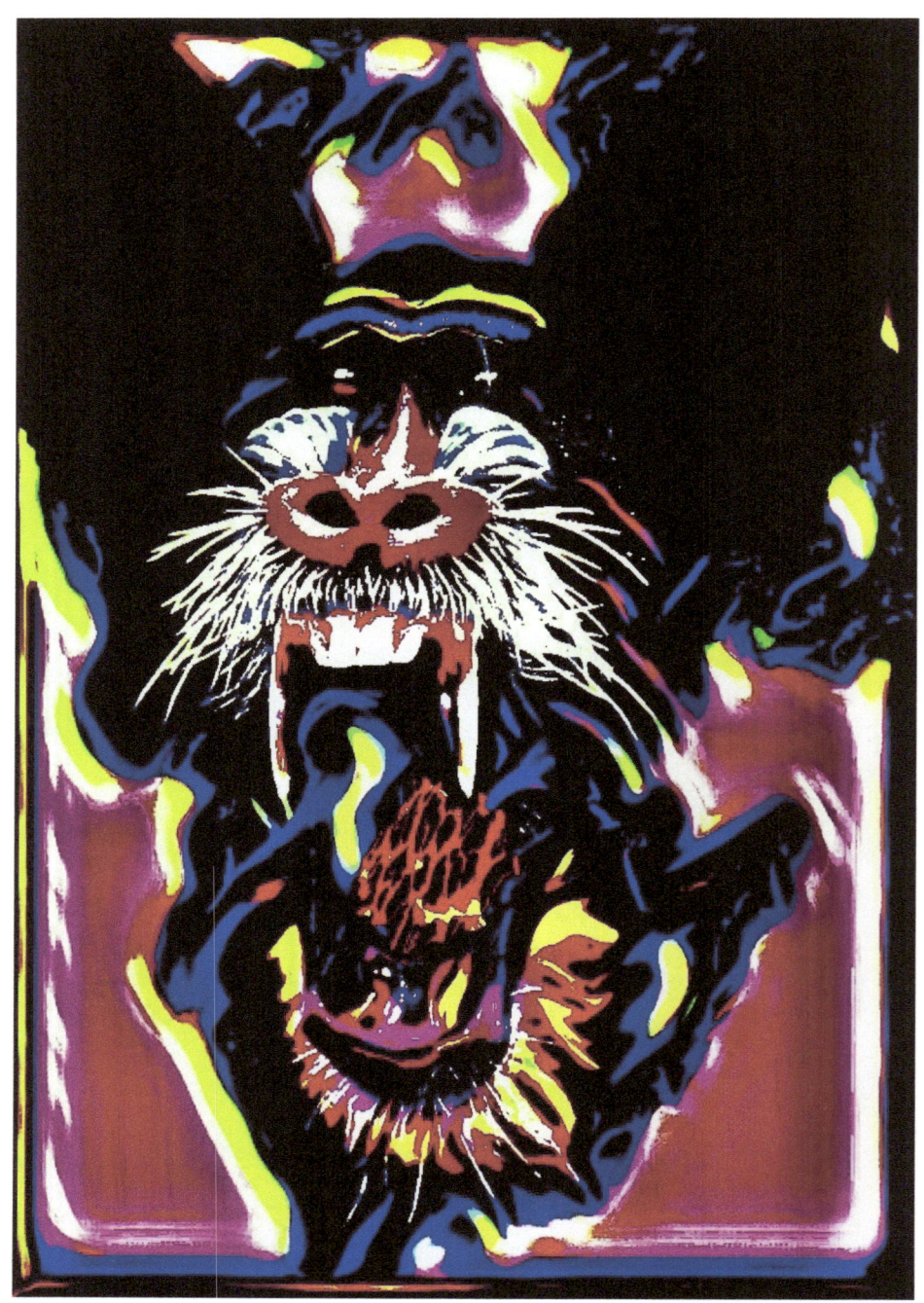

A blast from the marrow,

Outis: A Nursing Elegy

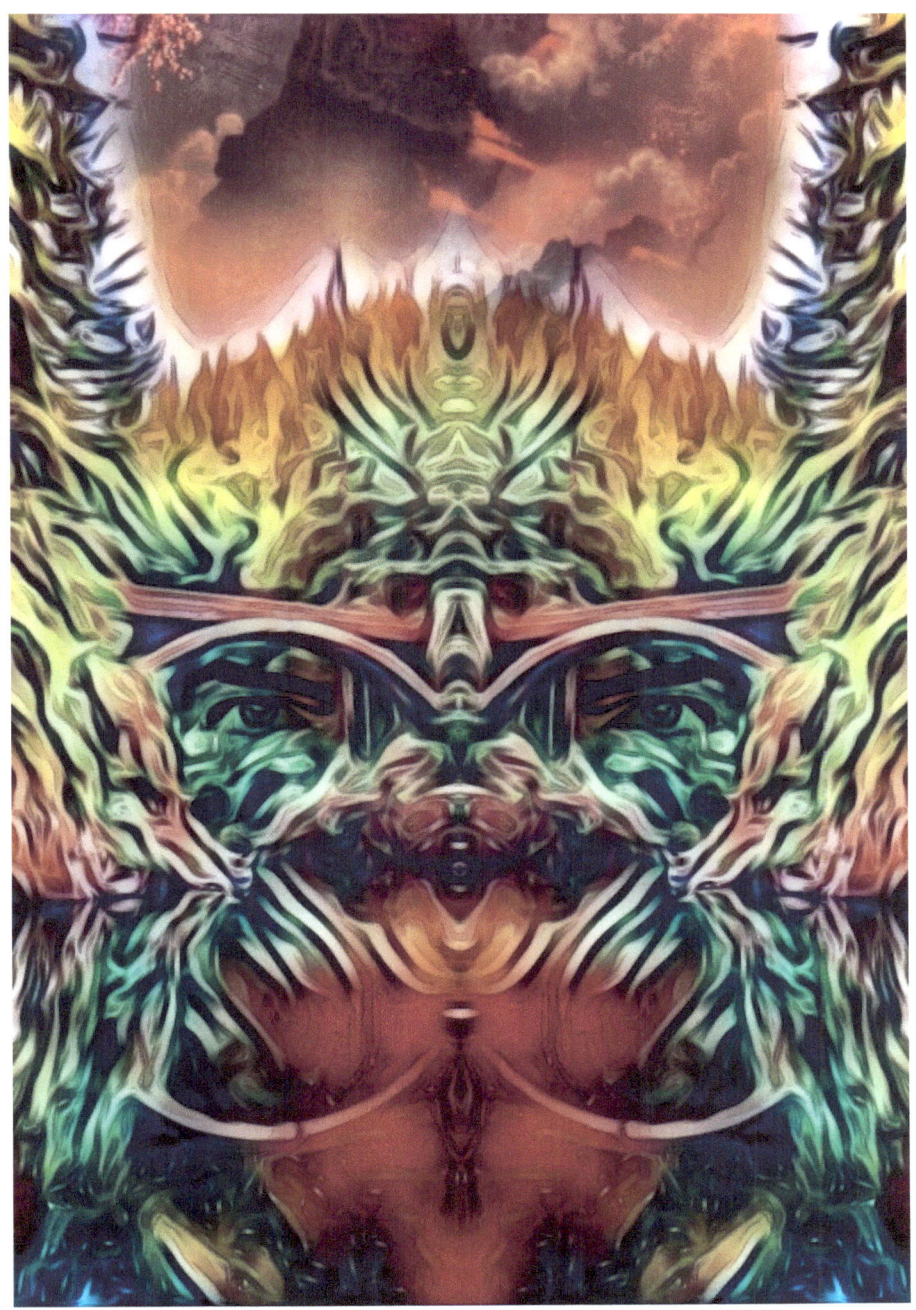

A sunset at morning-

Outis: A Nursing Elegy

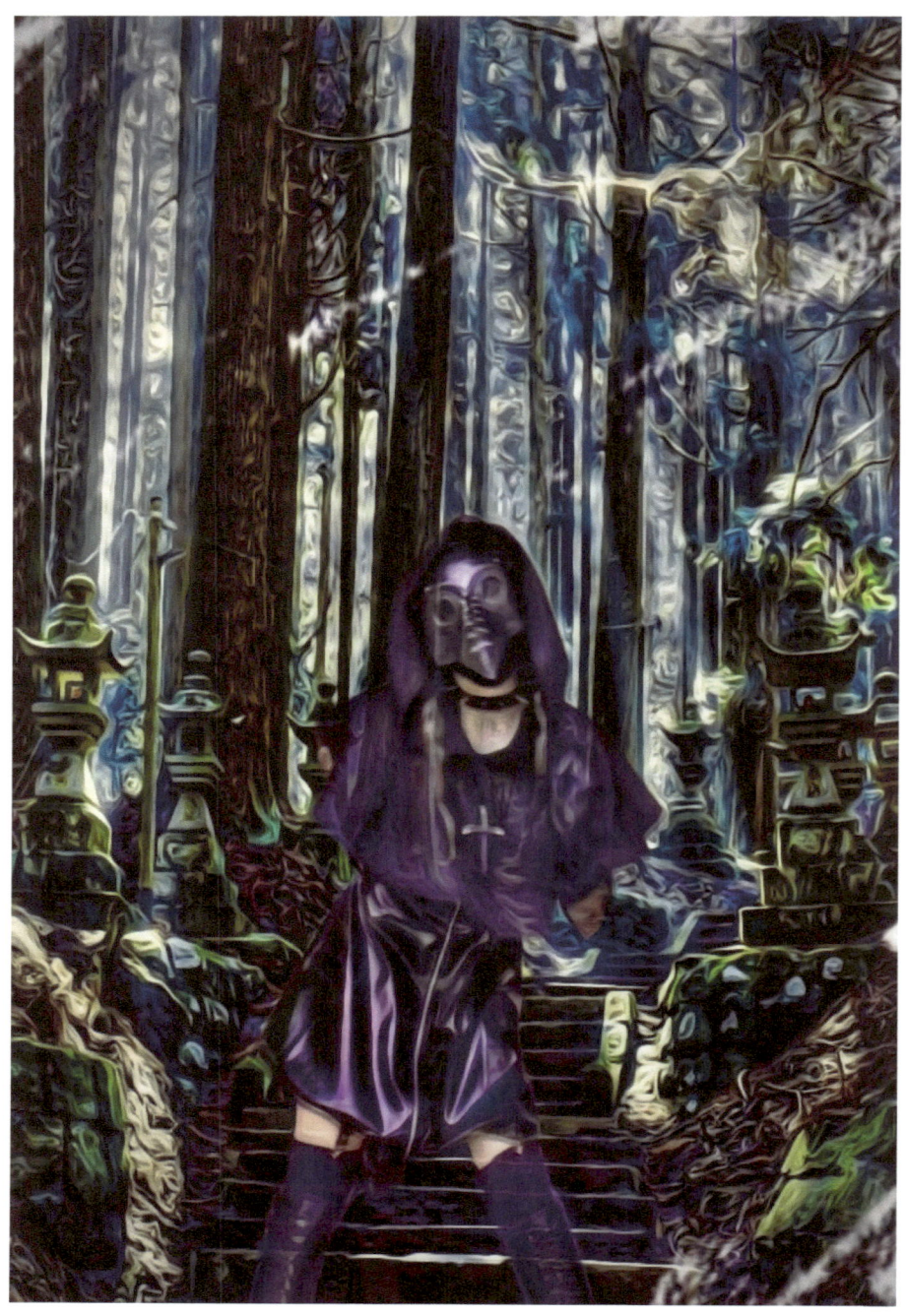

Imagery of nursing -

Outis: A Nursing Elegy

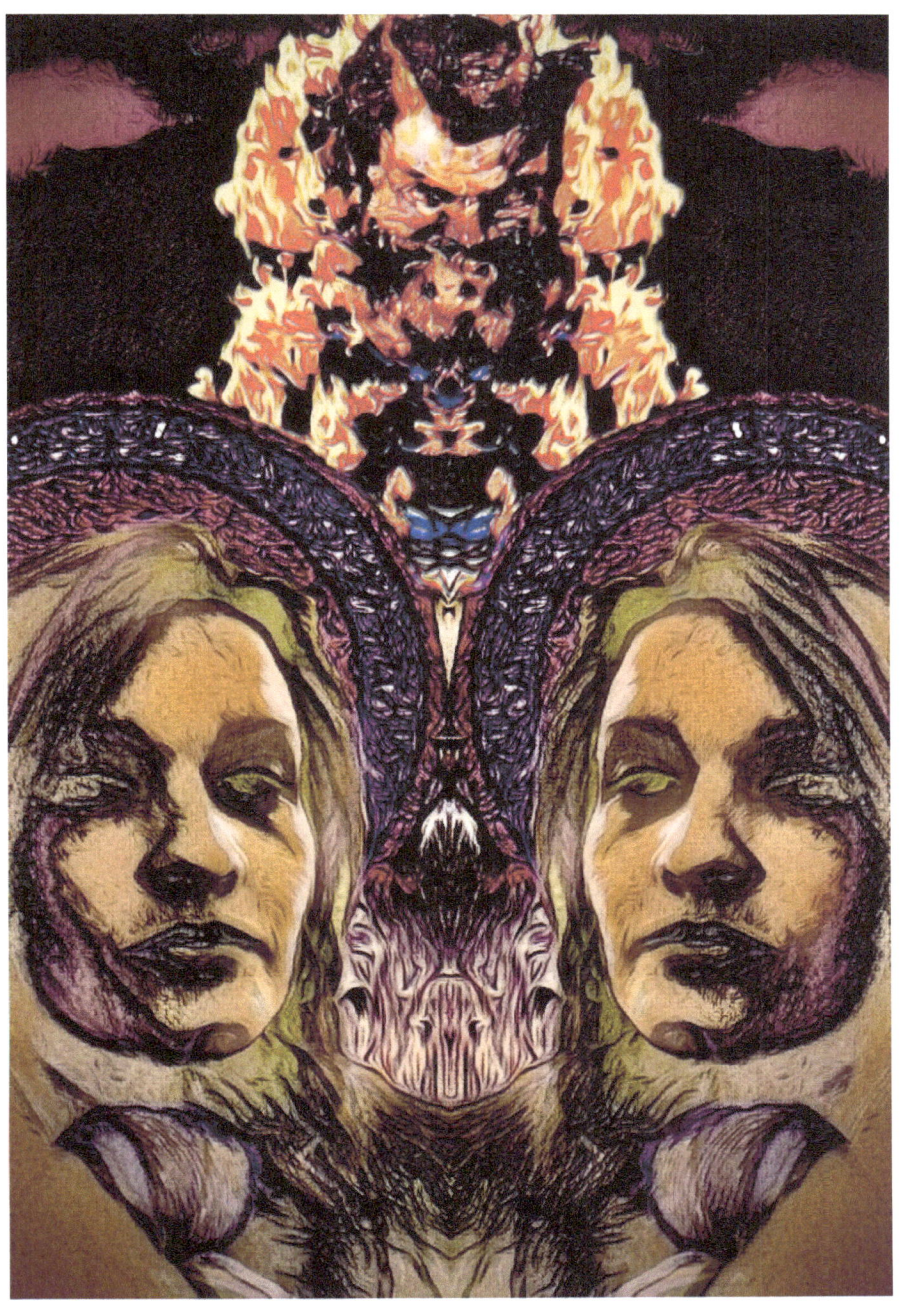

Mercy among torture-

Outis: A Nursing Elegy

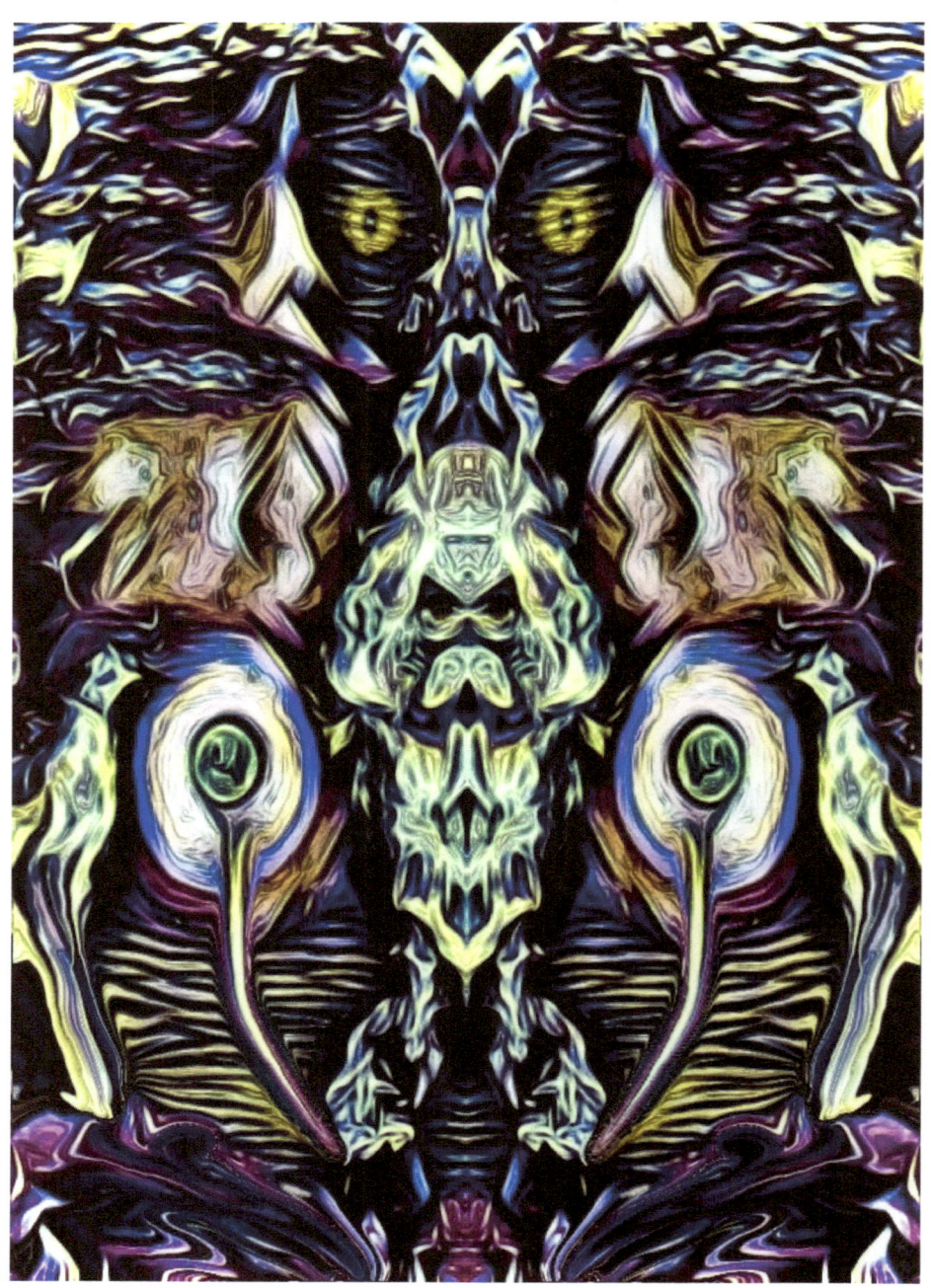

Bells of warning-

Outis: A Nursing Elegy

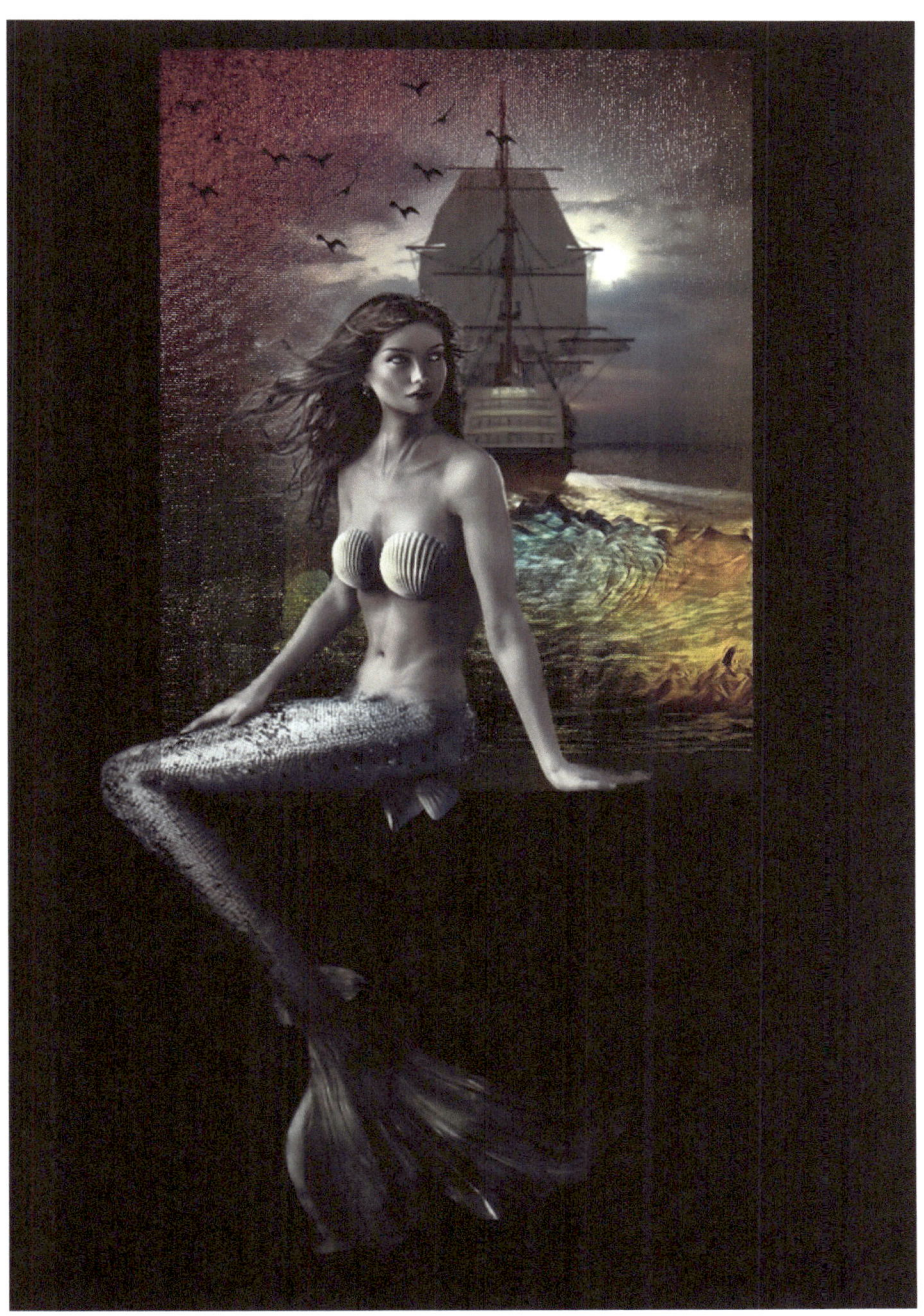

The Siren-surge of mourning-

Outis: A Nursing Elegy

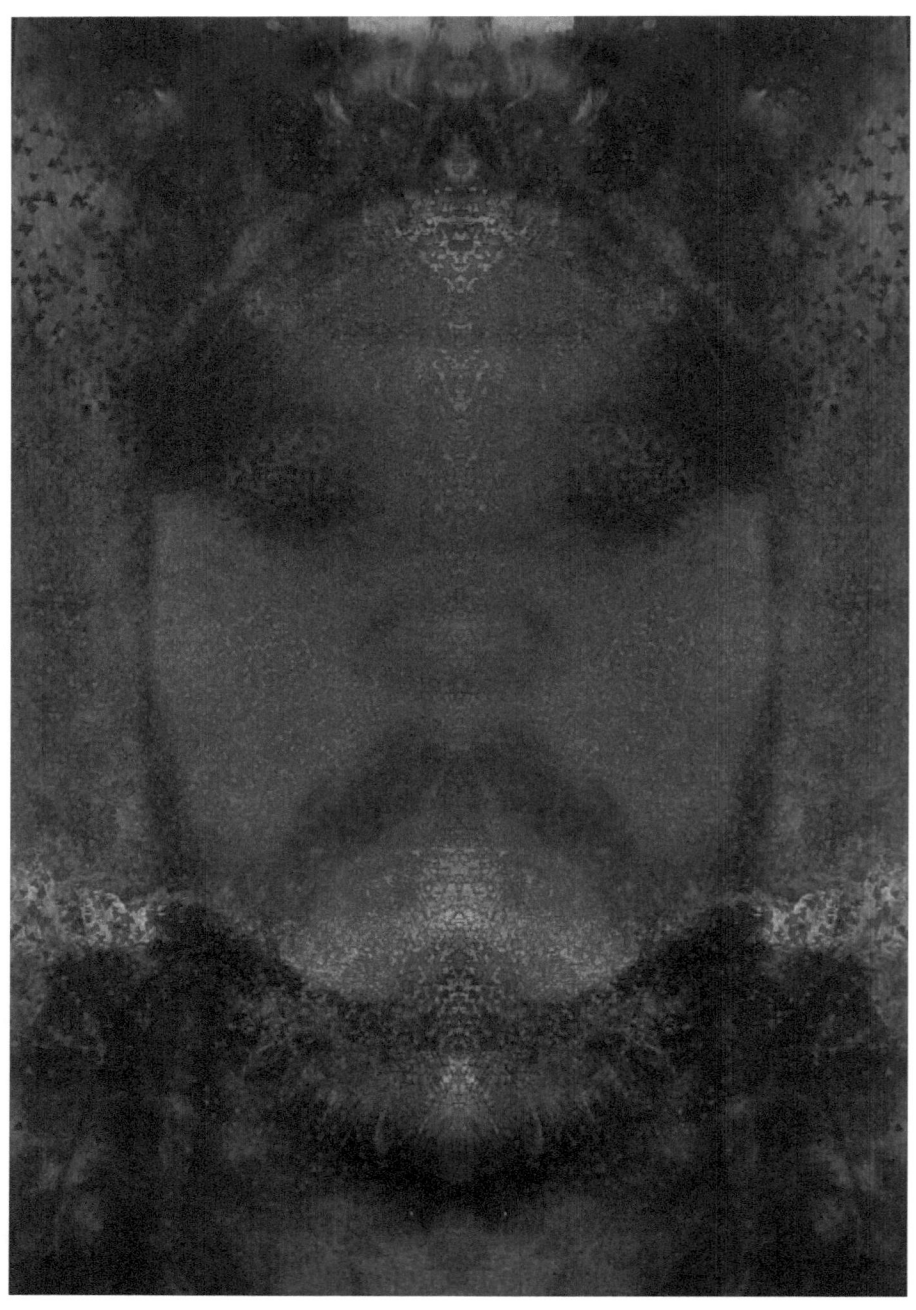

An odyssey of the "No One" will sail on by

Outis: A Nursing Elegy

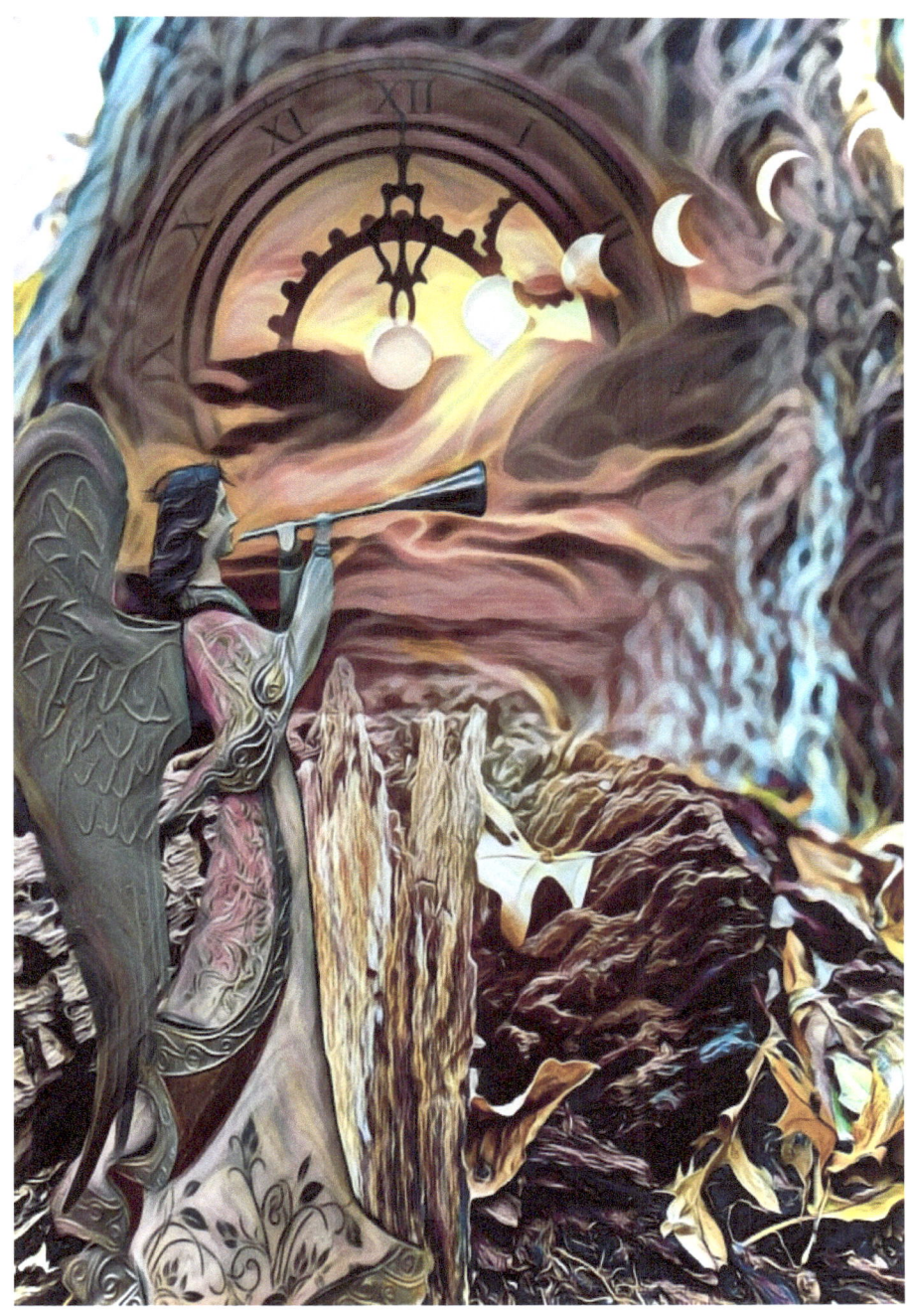

In the rebellion against the fate of who'll die.

Outis: A Nursing Elegy

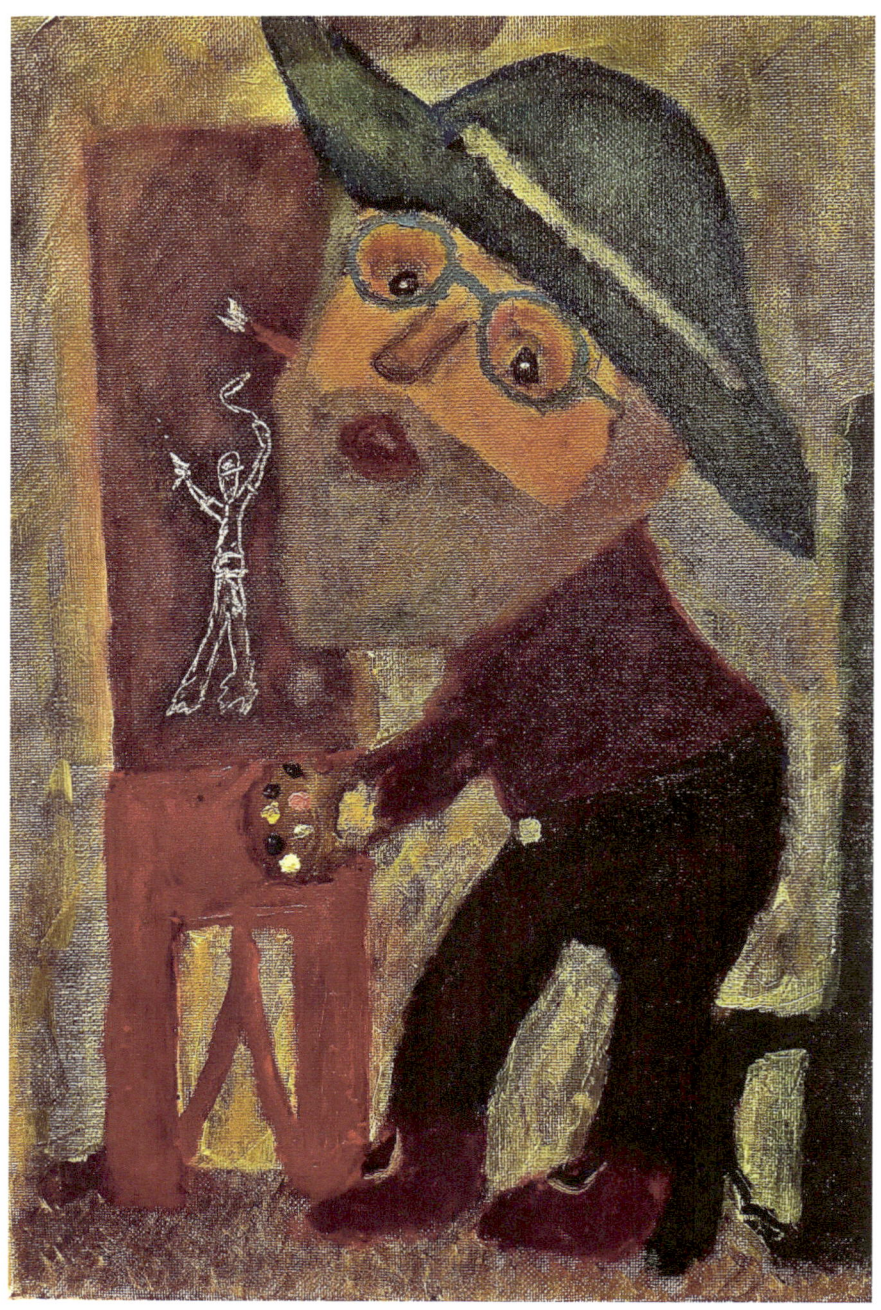

Outis: A Nursing Elegy

Outis

I.

The autumn rain dripping from the shedding boughs
Waving to and fro from winds whirling up a cold-
A haiku to decipher nature's fickle vows.

Home-lost travelers tread through the trials of trails.
Tales tallied to tell to those that never patrolled
Like a ship with no sails among the gush of gales.

Winding breezes winnow through the harvest of grain. . .
Haystacks dance upon stubble-fields with hedge witches. . .
Breaths conspire, exhale the sacred name to a pain,

The ache of change. . . Spring promises broken by truth. . .
All doesn't bloom for beauty or live out its riches.
The sickness of youth can fester from well-dug roots

While petals suffocate in the howling of storms
And the thorns can draw fresh blood from the plucking mourns.

Outis: A Nursing Elegy

II.

The lilacs, in full bloom, cut short for grief's display:
A symbol that's seen but not always understood;
The perennial destined to return someday,

Not as the resurrection of flower and stem
But as the legacy of a root that withstood
Frozen enrapture of a December condemn.

True death comes not in the reap to those who see prime;
It is when decay settles upon the blossoms
That is when the passing becomes noted in time.

To lovers of essence, the presence lingers on
Like the soft echoing trills of woodland oscines;
Life lives on in life, even when todays are gone,

To be the lightning flash, not the thunder after:
The eternity now, mortality later.

Outis: A Nursing Elegy

III.

Born to a fate of death, life follows scripts of chance.
Cruel and unfair, the world offers no place to hide.
A suffering romances those that takes a stance.

Those that aim to please earns a hollowness in time.
Oblivion awaits those that blacken eyes of pry.
Martyr, libertine or hermit- all fall in their climb.

Fame is like breath- known today, forgotten tomorrow.
Rows of withered gravestones, markers for rotten bones:
Testaments of purpose, memories of sorrow.

How the-dead-once-lived continues to throb in bloodstreams
As ghosts of rhythm, the architects of hormones. . .
The souls that haunt the mystic ancestry of dreams.

A shifting shade in mood colors all perception;
Let them haunt you in the passion of expression.

Outis: A Nursing Elegy

IV:

The stormy mist and frost kiss on fresh-fallen leaves.
The moaning breeze cracking the shriveled tree fingers.
Nature manifests metaphors for those that grieve . . .

What is there for those who know the passing spirits
But not how the departed lived? How death lingers
In beds, in rooms that other souls must inherit.

Names fade from consciousness. - The fates become destined. -
While the life-uprising against death soldiers on.
Then a haunting flashes those of final blessings-

The defeat of knowing, the gasp of agony-
(Breaths of truths no one can divulge into a song.) -
To shed light on tragedies of reality:

Those that witness can only own experience.
One must decide if that's a curse or providence.

Outis: A Nursing Elegy

V.

The winds of grief whistle through the reeds of requiem.
Summer leaves become autumn gold and then take leave.
The winter-today hardens phantoms of ransom. . .

The charlatans try to ensure you in their wares
To become a lotus eater that never grieves
The war fallen and those causes left unaware.

And, although we are never found, we are not lost. . .
A loneliness among the beauty of nature,
The odd shift in seasonal patterns- that's the cost.

A blast from the marrow, a sunset at morning-
Imagery of nursing - mercy among torture-
Bells of warning- the Siren-surge of mourning-

An odyssey of the "No One" will sail on by
In the rebellion against the fate of who'll die.

www.ingramcontent.com/pod-product-compliance
Lightning Source LLC
Chambersburg PA
CBHW040318220526
45473CB00009B/2482